Listen with the Heart

RELATIONSHIPS AND HEARING LOSS

Listen with the Heart

RELATIONSHIPS AND
HEARING LOSS

Michael A. Harvey

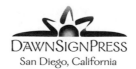

DawnSignPress
San Diego, California

Producer: Joe Dannis
Manufactured in the United States of America
Published by DawnSignPress

The information contained in this book is intended to be educational and not for diagnosis, prescription, or treatment of health disorders, whatsoever. This information should not replace competent medical care. The Author and Publisher are in no way liable for any use or misuse of the information.

Library of Congress Cataloging-in-Publication Data

Harvey, Michael A.
   Listen with the heart : relationships and hearing loss / Michael A. Harvey.
     p. cm.
   Includes bibliographical references.
   ISBN-13: 978-1-58121-019-4 (alk. paper)
   ISBN-10: 1-58121-019-1 (alk. paper)
   1. Hearing impaired—United States—Family relationships—Case studies. 2. Hearing impaired—United States—Psychology—Case studies. 3. Postlingual deafness—United States—Psychological aspects—Case studies. 4. Family psychotherapy—United States—Case studies.   I. Title.

HV2545 .H38 2001
362.4'23'0973—dc21

2001028228

10   9   8   7   6   5   4   3   2

For Janet, Allison, and Emily

On the Cover

Since the beginning of time relationships have been the most important hallmarks in people's lives. The "circle of friends" on the cover honors the closeness of those who gather in community in the hope that light and wisdom will grow out of their bond.

Acknowledgments

As I did in *Odyssey of Hearing Loss: Tales of Triumph,* I would like to begin by express my deep gratitude to the storytellers in this book. I hope I have done justice to narrating what transpired between us. Naturally, the names and details of each tale have been changed to protect confidentiality.

Marylyn Howe read, and often re-read, every word of *Listen with the Heart: Relationships and Hearing Loss* and provided her usual erudite feedback. She is a lasting friend and collaborator over the years for which I remain extremely grateful. My father, Harmond Harvey, offered helpful feedback, replete with a slew of grammatical corrections. Similarly, my mother, Barbara Hamburg, volunteered invaluable suggestions for increasing the book's interest and clarity while also correcting my grammar. Someday I hope to master the "I/me" challenge.

Many thanks to Richard Carmen, Roger Freeman, Pamela Gunther, Lisa Kaye, Marilyn Neault and Susan Rezen for their review of the book and helpful input. I also want to acknowledge people whose influences are present in this book: Ben Bahan, Hank Berman, Fran Demiany, Mike Finneran, Neil Glickman, Sanjay Gulati, Bob Hoffmeister, Gillian Kerr, Larry Kushner, Jeff Lewis, Steve Nover, Marie Philip, and Bob Pollard.

To Barbara Kelly, editor of *Hearing Loss,* for her support over the years, I give my thanks. It has been an honor to publish some of my work in the SHHH journal and also to answer readers' questions in the monthly column, "What's On Your Mind?"

It continues to be a pleasure working DawnSignPress. Many thanks to Joe Dannis for his support. As Rebecca Ryan did with *Odyssey*, I very much appreciate the dedication and care that she took with the production of this book. It has been a fun and easy collaboration. I am very grateful for the detailed and constructive editorial feedback from Kirsten Chrisman. Her comments on organization, style, presentation, and clarity were invaluable. Also many thanks to Barry Howland for his steadfast marketing efforts.

In one way or another, this book is a testament to the magic and work of intimacy. Here I owe the deepest gratitude to my wife, Janet Harvey, for the love, support, and guidance that she gives me and my children, Allison and Emily. We are unbelievably lucky. To Alli and Emily, I am thankful for the lessons of love and parenting they teach me, and that they allow me to teach them. Those life-long relationship lessons are the primary subject of this book.

Finally, much of the gratification I get from writing is from dialogue with readers. It would be my pleasure to respond to anyone who emails me at feedback@dawnsign.com (mention the book title in the subject line).

Contents

Introduction

Shared joys are doubled; shared sorrows are halved.
—English saying[1]

Hearing loss does not just affect an individual, but also one's family and friends. This book is a testament to those relationships. It contains true stories from my psychotherapy practice with individuals, couples, and families where there is a person (or persons) with hearing loss.[a] These tales portray how psychological, social, and spiritual influences shape one's experience of hearing loss and that of significant others. While at first glance these influences appear hopelessly entangled, the therapeutic dialogue serves to clarify their complexity.

A journalist was once asked, "How do you know when you are in a crisis?" His response was, "It's when questions arise that can't be answered."[2] There are an infinite number of questions that persons with acquired hearing loss are compelled to answer: e.g., "Why me?"; "What do I do now?"; "Who are my real friends?"; "How do I reconcile with God?" Indeed, the storytellers in this book described their *crises* of hearing loss. As Bill, in Overcoming Isolation

---

a. Naturally, the names and details of these tales have been changed to maintain confidentiality.

and Despair (Chapter 8) put it, "My becoming deaf is an utterly overwhelming and terrifying experience!"

Some readers may object that the *crisis* of "hearing loss" as described here seems negative and derogatory. But I don't think the matter is so simple. In my previous book, *Odyssey of Hearing Loss: Tales of Triumph,* I discussed how crises have a way of not only crushing but also strengthening the human spirit. In fact, when written in Chinese, the word "crisis" is composed of two characters. One represents danger, and the other represents opportunity.

I have been impressed with the transformative power of *relationships* to help those with hearing loss avoid the danger and find the opportunity. Each person portrayed in this book teaches us how when one shares with an intimate–other the struggle to reconcile the "questions that can't be answered," a special kind of wisdom can be achieved, not only for the person with the hearing loss but for everyone involved.

Participants in an intimate relationship are able to listen, not only with their heads, but with their hearts; they listen not only to the words, but seek to empathize with the other's experience; to *imagine* the inner workings of their psyche, to "listen intently to the urgent whisperings of another person's soul. *Who are you? What do you feel? What do you think? What means the most to you?*"[3] Carolyn, the hearing spouse of a man who suffered traumatic hearing loss (see Chapter 6, Vicarious Hearing Loss: A Spouse's Tale), learned a universal lesson: when we deeply connect with another human being in crisis, we are simultaneously, ever so subtly, changed ourselves. Her empathy with her husband catalyzed both his and her own psychological transformation.

The reader will find much in this book that is applicable to losses other than of hearing: often there is grieving, impact on self-esteem, the challenges of dealing with reactions of significant others, often conflicting professional guidance, and spiritual crises. At the same time, however, the stories chronicle many unique challenges of hearing loss, largely having to do with communication, self-identity, and interpersonal relationships.

My current emphasis on relationships at first may sound like a repetition of one of my previous books, *Psychotherapy with Deaf and Hard-of-Hearing Persons: A Systemic Model,* but that book was written in technical jargon for mental health professionals. Although the current book covers some of the same territory, I wrote it in a user-friendly, story-telling format. It is therefore accessible to a much wider audience, including spouses, children, parents, friends, extended family members, interested laypersons, and professionals. On my part, I've found that storytelling is often more instructive and fun to write than technical text.

A word about terminology: Throughout this book, I use the term "hearing loss" instead of Deaf deliberately. There are many members of the Deaf community who do not view themselves as having a disability or crisis of hearing loss, but rather as being proud members of a community, a culture, a linguistic minority.[b] However, the stories in this book are principally about those who have defined themselves from an audiological perspective as having experienced a reduction in or loss of hearing. They have experienced a loss of something they had taken for granted: like music, engaging in "pillow talk" with their partners, or hearing their children's voices. Rather than identify with the Deaf community and Deaf culture, they label themselves as having an "acquired hearing loss," as "hard-of-hearing," "late-deafened," "hearing-impaired," or as "deaf." Most use English as their primary language—not a signed language.

One exception is Debbie in Chapter 7, Beyond the Tug-of-War. Born with a profound hearing loss, she wants no part of the hearing

---

b. The lowercase **d**eaf refers to those who, from a audiological perspective, view themselves as having a profound hearing loss but who choose *not* to be culturally Deaf. **D**eaf (with a capital D) refers to culturally Deaf people.

world, even if, in her words, she could "become one of them." She does not define herself as disabled, but rather as part of the Deaf community. However, her husband, Jim, who has a progressive hearing loss, wears hearing aids and would jump at the chance to take a magic pill to regain his hearing. He is considering getting a cochlear implant. At Jim's request, Debbie accompanies him to the Association of Late-Deafened Adults or Self-Help for the Hard-of-Hearing conventions. At Debbie's request, Jim accompanies her to the National Association of the Deaf conventions.

There are boundless opportunities to "listen with the heart" in the context of relationships involving hearing loss, as it deeply affects loved ones and significant others. Ultimately there is always too much to say, too many feelings to share! It was Virginia Satir, a well-known family therapist, who said that when one member of a system is in crisis, each and every other member is also in crisis.[4] Thus, those who have an intimate relationship with the person who has a hearing loss share with him or her the potential for danger and opportunity.

Listen with the Heart: Relationships and Hearing Loss chronicles the psychological, social, and spiritual effects of hearing loss on an individual and on those surrounding persons. As we become privy to their intimate sharing of joy and sorrow with each other and with me as their psychotherapist, we marvel at the transformative power of relationships, how each partner has unparalleled opportunities to grow in profound and often unpredictable ways.

Notes

1. Frank, J. R. (1999). *Quotations dictionary.* New York: Random House.
2. Kapuscinski, R. (1985). *A Warsaw diary,* No. 15. Cambridge, England: Granta.
3. Ciaramicoli, A. P., & Ketcham, K. (2000). *The power of empathy: A practical guide to creating intimacy, self-understanding and love.* New York: Dutton.
4. Satir, V. (1972). *Peoplemaking.* Palo Alto, CA: Science and Behavior Books.

CHAPTER 1

Mourning My Mother, Welcoming My Family

"I wish I had understood the eulogy," Diane sighed. "I hadn't seen my brother cry since he was a young boy when he was in a sports accident. Boy stuff. But, as a grown man, Peter stood at the altar bawling his eyes out! He was eulogizing my mother."

Diane and I had been meeting for several months. As a toddler, she was first diagnosed as having a moderate hearing loss, cause unknown. However, it had become noticeably worse about four years ago at the age of 47, leaving her with minimal useable hearing. Until now, our psychotherapy sessions had focused on her handling feelings of alienation caused by lack of accommodations at work and the withdrawal of those whom she had considered dear friends.

Today we would discuss another alienating experience: her mother's funeral.

"The church was a huge echo chamber I was trapped inside," was Diane's deliberately worded summary statement. She had obviously spent much time choosing the precise descriptors that would do justice to her traumatic ordeal. She gazed upward as if to move time backward one-half year to when her mother had passed away. She elaborated: "I was bombarded by noise all around me—by muffled and distorted echoes, rumbles of clatter. My hearing aids only made them louder and more piercing. By the time the service was over, I had a splitting headache. So much for a sacred ritual."

Her sarcasm masked her feelings of helpless victimization and betrayal. Any comfort and sacredness were stolen from her and replaced with torture. One question was how and why did it happen?

The physical environment was an obvious culprit. Diane was describing a common frustration of hearing-aid users: namely, that a hearing aid by itself, without an additional assistive listening device, often amplifies background noise as well as the sound that one is attempting to focus on. This problem is particularly acute in poor acoustic environments in which there is an unacceptable *signal to noise ratio* and *reverberation.*

The signal to noise ratio refers to the level of background noise that interferes with one's ability to understand speech. According to audiologists, the ratio should be at least 20 dB: the speaker's voice should be at least 20 dB louder than any background noise.[1] Reverberation refers to the sound that reflects off the walls, ceiling, floor, and objects in the room. If the reflected sound (or echo) arrives immediately after the initial sound, it overlaps and does not cause excessive distortion. A reverberation time of no greater than 0.5 seconds is an acceptable standard.[2]

Carpeting, drapery, low ceilings and acoustical ceiling tiles are required to achieve these levels. The church, however—with its granite floor, stained glass windows, and high, vaulted ceiling—was anything *but* acoustically manageable for Diane. Instead, it had become an *echo chamber.*

"Why didn't you request that the people who spoke, like Peter, use some kind of assistive listening device—like an FM or infrared loop system?" I asked.

"My poor father and family had enough to worry about without having to get an FM system hookup, so I said nothing." She sighed again and stared blankly out my office window.

I wondered about the historical context in which Diane's decision to "say nothing" was embedded. Was she typically passive and overaccommodating, perhaps not wishing to make trouble or inconvenience anyone? Was she embarrassed to assert her audiological needs with her family? Did they overtly or covertly dismiss her needs? Or perhaps Diane used the "echo chamber" to hide or distance herself from her family, like a kind of psychological citadel? Many questions.

I simply asked her to tell me more about why she said nothing.

"Although my Mom and Dad always told me to ask them to repeat what people said, I noticed how it would become annoying to them, particularly after the second or third time. They didn't have to say anything—I knew! My brothers and sisters, however, were more direct; they would say 'it's nothing important' or 'what's it to you?' It's funny that I often couldn't understand many of their conversations, but their sighs and rebuffs were always loud and clear to me. At my mom's funeral, I didn't want to be the cause *once again* of anyone's sighs."

"If it's not too much bother, I'd like to understand my mother's eulogy," I replied, admittedly with a sarcastic edge to my voice.

"Yeah, something like that," she said. Diane understood my sarcasm.

"Tell me about you and your mother," I said.

"I was the first to learn about the pinkish toilet water," she began. "By mistake, I walked in the bathroom after my mother had urinated. There was blood in the toilet! It would be several days until she finally told her doctor. As the middle of two brothers and two sisters, I was always the closest to her. She confided in me about almost everything, even to the point that it made my siblings resentful.

"I had the dubious status of being the special needs kid in the family," she said. "My mom went to endless school meetings, audiology appointments, doctors, and speech therapists—all because of me. But she usually did it lovingly and never made me feel guilty or undeserving. She was a wonderful advocate and a wonderful mother."

Her voice cracked and tears came to her eyes. She had lost not only her mother but her advocate and best friend. I asked her about her relationship with other family members.

"My dad was different. He delegated the task of comforting me to my mom by sending her into my bedroom when I was sad. He was a good manager in that way. I always got the feeling that he was a bit scared of me, that he didn't know quite what to do. And my brothers and sisters—they've never gotten over their resentment about what a bloody distraction I was. Once my brother, Peter, was finally going to get a trombone; he was thrilled until my parents rescinded their promise. They would have to buy me new hearing aids instead."

Diane shook her head and continued, "Just the other day, my sister, Jill, was reminiscing to me how her needs never quite seemed important enough to Mom: 'Nothing, *absolutely nothing,* was a match against your IEP (Individualized Educational Plan),' Jill told me. 'Not my gymnastics, ballet, debating team, school dances; NOTHING! If only the rest of us had IEPs, too.'

"Jill was smiling, though," Diane was quick to point out. "As adults, we laugh about all of that now. We're much closer; her resentment is past-tense."

I sensed that Diane opened the door to exploring uncharted territory—her family's resentment toward her—only to push everything back in the "past tense." My task was to gently nudge her forward.

"Then how was it that they helped to isolate you at your mother's funeral?" I asked. So much for gentle nudges, I thought.

"What do you mean?"

This time I was more careful. "You know, opposite emotions, like resentment and appreciation, love and anger, can go together. Maybe your family can authentically laugh about old resentments; but old wounds have a habit of sometimes reappearing in the present with their original venom, particularly during family crises. I know you didn't feel comfortable, in your words, 'being the cause of anybody's sighs at your mom's funeral.' But on the other hand, no-body in your family offered to help make it accessible to you. So you ended up not understanding the eulogy of your mother, the one who had given you the most attention!"

"It is ironic, isn't it?" Diane said.

"Irony has its hidden reasons," I replied. I wanted to keep the door of past/present resentments open for further exploration. However, Diane's attention was focused elsewhere. I asked her what she was thinking.

"Cancer is a slow, slow death," Diane reminisced, in reference to her mother. "Her hair thinned out, then turned a whitish gray, and then fell on her sheets. Rashes spread all over her body. Right before my eyes, as weeks and months trudged forward, my mom shriveled down from 210 to finally 90 pounds! Out of her body came a corpse. It was a *torturous execution!*" Diane grimaced.

It felt important that Diane had also used the word "torture" to describe her ordeal at the church. But we would explore that later. Now only her mother's lurid death permeated our discussion. I re-called author Ivan Illich's wish that *"he wouldn't die of some disease. Instead, he wanted to die of death."*[3] His wish finally made sense to me upon hearing Diane's story. I nodded my head and asked her to continue.

"I visited her at the hospice—where she spent the last several weeks of her life—at least four or five times a week, if not more. I didn't hesitate about taking an extended leave of absence from work; it was the right thing to do. In a second of clarity my priorities be-came clear. There would be hundreds of business opportunities; my mother would die only once."

A profound and refreshing attitude, I thought.

"When I sat at her bedside—just the two of us, holding hands—we would reminisce about old, joyful times: when she met my first boyfriend or when she gave me endless preparatory lectures for when I would begin my period (it would be several years later); the first time I baked banana bread and used baking soda instead of baking powder; and when she let me have a sip of beer without Dad knowing. I wanted us to cherish every remaining moment we had; to laugh, to cry, to be close—to make every moment of our time together last forever.

"I tried to give her hope. We would pray and beg the doctors to bestow to us even a minute possibility of a recovery, a medical miracle. But she was obviously slipping away. It was a hell of a struggle to fight back my tears. I barely did it." Diane's lips trembled, not so much with sadness but with an intensity that became clear only upon her next sentence: "*But it was no struggle at all to understand her!*" Diane's countenance quickly changed, and her voice now had more emphasis. "Each and every word on her lips was crystal clear!"

"How did it go when your family came to visit her?" I asked.

"I instantly became the handicapped, hearing-impaired, inept kid again," she quickly responded, now in a lower, more frail voice. Like an on-off switch. Competent versus incompetent. Connected versus disconnected.

"All of us—my sister and her husband and two kids, my brother, his wife and new baby, et cetera—would sit in a sort of circle around my mother's bed. I sat on the periphery. The children would get restless and cranky; then they would run around the room, knocking things over and making a racket. That's how the visit would go."

"And what was that like for you?" I asked.

"Like a glass bubble was put over me. I could see everybody clearly but could understand hardly a word. Loud clatter!"

"And what did you do?"

"I did the best I could."

"Did you get headaches?" That was one effect of the echo chamber at her mother's funeral.

"Yeah. I would get migraines that sometimes lasted for hours!"

"Did anyone notice or ask how you were doing?"

"No," Diane replied. "I don't know why, but no one asked." She looked down toward the floor in shame.

"Love and resentment can cohabitate," I said, referring back to how past resentments tend to reappear in families. It was as if her siblings were getting back at Diane for all the attention that her mother had given her during their childhood. Payback time. There is a saying attributed to Mahatma Gandhi: "If you follow the old code of justice—an eye for an eye and a tooth for a tooth—you end up with a blind and toothless world."[4] Payback doesn't work.

I asked Diane about inviting her father and some of her siblings to one of our sessions, so I could understand the family background more. Moreover, as an important aside, her mother's one-year memorial service was scheduled for six months from now and I wanted to help avoid a repetition of Diane's echo chamber entrapment. She readily agreed. At her suggestion, we would begin with her father, her sister, Jill, and her brother, Peter, who had eulogized their mother about six months ago.

I asked her the crucial question: "How can we make it so communication is accessible for you during our meeting?" For a group conversation, hearing-aids would not be adequate as they were for our individual, one-to-one meetings.

She seemed taken aback somewhat, as if she had never considered that question in the context of her family and was surprised that I had asked it. After a moment, she replied somewhat tentatively, "Well, I do have a portable microphone apparatus."

"Uh huh." I prompted her.

"I guess I can bring it in," she conceded. Her hesitancy was apparent.

"Good!" was my simple response. I could have, and perhaps should have, explored her ambivalence which undoubtedly related back to family dynamics. But we were out of time and I didn't want to lose the momentum of her having agreed to a family meeting.

Two weeks later, Diane, Jill, Peter, and their father, Larry, entered my office. After we exchanged miscellaneous pleasantries and a mutual irritation with the local road construction, I matter-of-factly asked Diane to explain how the portable FM system worked. It was a standard, simple opening request, as we couldn't begin our meeting without ensuring accessible communication. Yet that simple objective was entangled in unspoken, emotional undercurrents. The first moments of our session would be both the most difficult and essential. At least for now, though, these undercurrents would remain implicit and unacknowledged.

Diane awkwardly demonstrated the use of the FM system and asked the three of them "if they wouldn't mind" passing the microphone to whomever was speaking. They were, I think, authentically accommodating and gracious but nevertheless looked somewhat put out. Perhaps it was my imagination, I thought.

A probe: "It certainly stilts the conversation a bit," I observed openly to the group. I passed the microphone half-way between them. Larry took it.

"It's no bother, really. The important thing is that Diane understands us," Larry responded.

I took the microphone. "That's much easier said than done. Talking one-at-a time and giving cues who's talking, for example, surely ruins many opportunities for spontaneous, quick jokes." It would be important not to oversimplify many years of entrenched family dynamics as completely resolvable solely by a technological aid. My other goal here was to avoid any appearance of siding with Diane against the others. As a hearing person myself, I can empathize with how artificial the communication process can sometimes feel when ensuring accessibility.

"It's no bother, really," was the response.

We spent the next few minutes reviewing standard communication rules, such as always being sure to pass the microphone to the respective speaker and speaking one at a time. Once they were clear and everyone agreed on the rules, we discussed some family history and events. Passing the microphone back and forth very much slowed down the fast-paced, talking-over-each-other, free-for-all competition that is characteristic among hearing persons. Moreover, this intervention served to keep Diane's communication needs in primary focus and to ensure that they were not usurped.

After a while, when I felt enough rapport with Jill, Peter, and Larry, I asked another essential question: "What was the funeral like for each of you?"

Jill and Larry both responded with versions of "it was very moving," "emotional," "Peter told a beautiful story," "it was what she would have wanted." Peter blushed.

"And what about you?" I asked Diane, admittedly as an impromptu act of putting her on the spot.

She, however, was ready. "You know damn well, Mike," Diane said. Now turning to face her family, she indicted them with "But you don't!"

After a pause, she regained her composure. Perhaps her accusatory outburst scared her. She continued in a softer, less angry but more self-depreciating tone. "I'm sorry, maybe I should have said something much earlier. I didn't want to be a bother, you know, like I was as a kid, always asking 'Whad'ya say? Whad'ya say?'"

"And the funeral?" I prompted her.

After taking a deep breath, she bravely recounted how her experience of the funeral was the opposite of beautiful and moving. She described instead the piercing thunder of sounds in the church echo chamber. This was the first time she had disclosed these traumatic memories to the three family members who sat in my office, now with their mouths open.

Moments passed. Finally, her father took the microphone and asked, "You mean you didn't understand any of the service?"

"I hadn't seen my brother cry since he was a kid," she said. "But I couldn't understand what he was saying." Her statement was almost verbatim what she had told me much earlier.

The room was silent. Everyone was absorbing and reconciling Diane's confirmation of conversational inaccessibility that they had denied for decades.

I broke the silence with one short phrase. "The solution is so simple but so damn complicated." I didn't intend to be cryptic, rather only to observe that Diane *could have* let them know that she found it impossible to understand what was being said about her mother and that someone *could have* just as easily asked. I was reminded of a colleague who joked, "People with anorexia simply should eat more, depressed people should smile." True, but not that simple.

"Would you like to hear Peter recount his eulogy?" I asked Diane.

Taken aback as if she had never given that possibility much thought, she tentatively responded with "Well, I guess so—sure."

"Peter, I know this is short notice. But would you, as best you can, give Diane a recap?"

"Uh, sure," he stammered as he was given the microphone. He looked somewhat embarrassed, perhaps because of what he had just heard from Diane and/or because I was putting him on the spot. Like Diane had done with me during another meeting, Peter paused and mentally moved time backward to when his mother had passed away. He, too, took a deep breath and began:

"I told my favorite story. One day when I was 8 years old, I was chosen to be the starting pitcher for the championship baseball game of the season. My friends were busy; and my dad's work had taken him out-of-town for several days. It was my mom who volunteered to help me practice. On a scorching hot Saturday morning, she crouched down at home plate for hours with her hands firmly in a catcher's mitt, catching my curve balls, sliders, and fast balls. She also gave me pitching tips. We won that game because of her. But I never said thank you. So I'll do it now. Better late than never. Thank you, Mom, if you're here listening to this. I love you."

Our eyes filled with tears. Diane made eye contact with Peter who gave her back a loving smile. It was a beautiful memory, I thought. And it opened another door.

I asked Peter how old he was when Diane's hearing loss was identified.

"It was shortly after my tenth birthday." Peter said.

"Before or after that championship baseball game?" I asked.

"After." I sensed that he knew exactly where I was going. Before I could ask the next question, he supplied the answer: "After we found out Diane had a hearing problem, Mom's time was spent at schools and doctors' appointments."

At that second, Jill nodded her head and muttered, "I miss her."

I asked Peter to pass Jill the microphone so that her comment would be accessible to Diane.

"Sorry," Diane said awkwardly, "but would you mind repeating what you said?"

Jill repeated her declaration into the microphone: "I miss Mom, I miss Mom a lot!"

"I miss her, too," Diane replied. They exchanged a tearful glance.

Whether or not Jill meant to avoid the sensitive subject of Diane's newly diagnosed hearing loss usurping Mom's attention, it was now Diane who took the lead in bringing us back on that difficult but important track. "I'm sorry I took Mom away from you [looking at Jill and Peter]. I didn't mean to. I was a kid."

This time Peter quickly intervened with "It was no one's fault; it just happened."

But Diane persevered: "I know that; but you've been angry, you've never told me but I've always sensed it. You had a right to be angry! You, too Jill; you, too, Dad."

The three of them needed no further explanation or coaxing, now affirming her perception by nodding their heads. It was Peter who provided the words: "You're right. We had been angry, probably without even realizing it. In some ways, I suppose, you getting your needs met as a kid meant us not getting ours met. There was only so much of Mom to go around, you know. But it doesn't have to be that way anymore." His voice was soft and tender.

Larry had been on the edge of his seat, taking in what was a long overdue discussion among his children. He, too, needed no prodding to speak. Into the microphone, he said "That's where you're wrong, Pete. It *didn't* have to be a win-lose proposition when you all were kids. In truth, we were all a bit scared—I certainly was—and I didn't have any idea what to do about Diane's hearing loss. Your mother being the fighter she was sort of jumped in and went to battle. I guess I relied on her too much; I could've done more. I let you kids down, and I'm really, really sorry. I'm just grateful and relieved that all of you turned out okay."

With flushed faces, the children nodded their heads, and Jill reached over and held her dad's hand. He fought back tears. Everyone fell silent.

Now our two-hour meeting was coming to an end. Interestingly, it was Larry—who, by his own admission, had remained disengaged over the years—who requested more family meetings. We scheduled three more sessions and planned to invite the remaining siblings.

Over the next couple of months, I met with the whole family: Larry and his six children. Our sessions routinely began by my prompting Diane to review communication rules and by my eliciting other family members' reactions. Only then would we focus on understanding how both the mother's death and Diane's hearing loss had changed things for this family.

It became increasingly clear that Diane's coming to terms with her mother's death was a multileveled endeavor. Initially, it required her to acknowledge how her hearing loss had, in part, defined their relationship. They had an intimacy that everyone envied. As much as Diane was shut out of her mother's funeral, she had been a privileged insider with her mother: a recipient of her advocacy efforts and a confidant to her hopes, dreams, and fears that she hadn't shared with the others.

On another level, Diane was also obliged to acknowledge how her hearing loss had helped mold her relationships with all other family members. Disengagement, resentment, envy, and compassion were frequent themes.

Finally, Diane learned how her hearing loss had influenced the larger family drama. The younger siblings vehemently fought for their mother's attention with a constant "whining about not getting enough." Diane recalled feeling that the tension represented more than just sibling rivalry, that, in fact, her siblings had been relegated to second place. Moreover, Larry had become disengaged and immobilized in reaction to Diane's hearing loss and family fighting. He withdrew not only from Diane, but from his other children and wife as well.

As Peter later said, "Dad wanted perfect children; he didn't know what to do with anything less than that." A familiar experience for many parents. It was a pity that he didn't realize that perfection comes only in fantasies, that bonding with your children necessarily means relishing what they become and coming to terms with what they fail to become.

Whereas the past is unalterable, the future is full of rich opportunities. One such opportunity would be the upcoming memorial service for their mother that, by this time, was scheduled in a couple of months. I had suggested to Diane that she meet with her audiologist to go over the logistics of various assistive listening devices for the memorial service. She already had her family's permission and blessings.

Diane, however, took one giant step forward on her own. She invited all five siblings and Dad to meet with her audiologist. They accepted. She later told me that the audiologist had specifically explained and demonstrated how an FM system worked, and, more generally, how the service could be made accessible for people who use hearing aids, including a discussion of signal to noise ratios, reverberation, etc. With obvious satisfaction and pride, Diane recalled her own response when the audiologist said to her, "This device may help you become involved in the ceremony somewhat better than before."

"I said to the audiologist that the FM system will help my family as much as it will help me; because if I'm part of their conversation, I can contribute to it. I can give something back."

Diane was right. *Assistive listening devices are as much for hearing persons as they are for those with a hearing loss.*

Diane and her family planning the logistics of her mom's memorial set the stage for dramatic changes of relationships—*a ripple of relational shifts*—to occur. With her dad, for example, Diane told me that "I noticed him withdrawing and acting overwhelmed like he tends to do. So I apologized for my making things even more difficult by needing special accommodations. He stopped everything, took me aside and said, 'Don't ever apologize for that again! Your mom isn't here to tell you it's okay to get your needs met; and she'll never be here to do that again. Now it's my turn. I should have said these things to you long ago.'"

There were sibling relational shifts as well. All five siblings split the cost of renting the FM system. Peter articulated their reason to Diane: "As kids we were *forced* to forgo certain things because of needing to spend money on you; now it's *our choice.* Yeah, it might stilt things a bit but I really want you to understand me, just like I want to understand you."

Diane was one of the scheduled speakers at the memorial service. Here is a segment from her memorial speech:

> Since our dear mother's death one year ago today, I've finally been able to say what I have always felt: that I stole her from my family. But I did this not out of malice, not even with awareness. But I didn't do it alone; the rest of family have courageously told me how they had helped. They were the accomplices. And Mom, too, was a willing participant. She gave me her love and support freely.
>
> To be honest though, I don't know if I would change the past even if I could. Her commitment to help me not become handicapped by my hearing loss gave me wonderful years at school and many wonderful childhood memories. I owe her for my life today. But her gift came with a cost.
>
> I've spent much of my life feeling guilty for what Mom had given me. You all lost a big part of her. Peter lost a pitching coach, Jill lost a dancing coach, and my Dad lost his wife. Robert, John, and Mary [her younger siblings] never even had the chance to get those gifts from Mom.
>
> Until recently, I sentenced myself for my supposed crime to a forced isolation from all of you who I love more than my words can express. I don't deserve that sentence, and neither do you. Our mother will always be with us in our hearts, as she is here with us today. And because of her death from

our physical world, we no longer have to compete for her attention. Her love and energy will now be in infinite abundance; it won't have to be divided up.

During the last months of her life, we took short walks every Sunday morning along the river. I'd pick her up early and she would pack a picnic lunch. When she was unable to walk, I'd push her in a wheelchair. That is where I still spend many Sunday mornings—walking with Mom. I talk to her, share intimacies, ask her for advice (last week I showed her a dress that I had bought). I tell her how much I love her. I thank her for what she has given me.

Won't you join us by the river?

Notes

1. Hawkins, D. B. (1990). "Amplification in the classroom." In J. Davis (ed.). *Our forgotten children: Hard-of-hearing pupils in the schools.* Washington DC: Self Help for Hard of Hearing People.
2. Hawkins, D. B. (1990). "Amplification in the classroom." In J. Davis (ed.). *Our forgotten children: Hard-of-hearing pupils in the schools.* Washington DC: Self Help for Hard of Hearing People.
3. Moore, T. (1992). *Care of the soul: A guide for cultivating depth and sacredness in everyday life.* New York: Harper Collins.
4. Johnson, R. A. (1991). *Owning your shadow.* San Francisco, CA: Harper.

CHAPTER 2

A Long Strange Trip

Sheila let out a sarcastic "hell if I know" when I asked what first attracted her to Jack. It seemed too long ago, buried under years of bitterness, resentment, hurt, and betrayal. Her confession exemplified a familiar principle of coupling: the more magic the falling in love—the "I know we just met, but I feel as though I already know you" phase—the more painful the inevitable downfall. The advantage of love at first sight is that it delays a second sight.

Before Jack could retaliate, I asked him, "What attracted you to Sheila?"

His response was pained, not angry as I had predicted. "She once had an inner beauty, a soft-spoken sensitivity to the world. Her inability to hear made her more intuitive; she picked up on cues that no one else noticed."

"Tell me more about her intuition."

"She intuited some of my deepest feelings and emotions, ones that even I didn't know I had. I would start a sentence, and she would complete it!"

"At that time, her deafness was an asset. In your mind, it made her more sensitive to your needs?" I asked.

"That's how it *was*," Jack said as he shook his head in resignation.

"You were a hell of a lot more sensitive back then, too!" Sheila interjected loud and clear. Having become profoundly deaf at the age of 14, as a result of meningitis, her speech was quite intelligible. She was more oriented to the hearing world, knew limited sign, and had only a few deaf acquaintances. She also had no difficulty understanding her husband's speech, which probably felt to her like a mixed blessing, I thought.

Jack did not respond. He was consumed grieving the loss of a seemingly idyllic union. He muttered, "It's come to this: having to go to a shrink!"

They had met on a nighttime cruise across Boston Harbor—a dark night, lit only by a full moon with a backdrop of stars. Jack recollected the magic of their courtship: "I never before felt so happy and fulfilled. Even one minute away from Sheila was unbearable! Everything was different: people I disliked seemed nicer, colors were brighter, food tasted better, and I even smelled flowers when there were none within miles!" Friends told him that he radiated a luminosity that was evident to anyone he encountered, family member or bank teller.

After shaking his head again, as if to acknowledge cherished but played-out memories long since passed, he made a final observation: "It was like being a child all over again."

Indeed, romantic love has been described as a return to an infantile, undifferentiated state of wholeness: a magical time when our parents filled us up, a state of bliss when our every wish and need was automatically gratified. When we fall in love, walls of isolation and self-consciousness no longer exist—only total innocence, eternal ecstasy. A dream come true. The end of our perpetual search for what we lost as children.

A problem: perpetual searches do not end. When we finally take our first objective look at our lover—typically soon after we make a life-long commitment to the relationship—we discover their warts and blemishes, deformities, flaws—all those negative traits that we had steadfastly refused to see.[1] Of course, on one level, their imperfections come as no surprise; our rational side knows our lover is not made of divine material. But, as psychologist Harvel Hendrix noted, the emergence of our lover's flaws nevertheless comes as a visceral shock, the ultimate betrayal, and thrusts us into the feelings of abandonment and outrage.

As a *life partner*, it suddenly is not enough that our lover be caring, witty, attractive, and fun loving. Now she or he has to satisfy a whole hierarchy of expectations, only some of which are conscious. Our partner must fulfill our unmet childhood needs, love us the way our parents never did, complement lost parts of ourselves, nurture us in consistent and loving ways, know our innermost thoughts and wishes, and be eternally available to us.[2] Easy to do, but only in the abstract.

Now turning to Sheila, I again asked her to "move time backward" and recall, as much as she could, what originally attracted her to Jack.

This time, she gave my question serious thought. "Well, I always assumed I would someday marry a deaf man; someone who would understand me and not put me down like so many hearing people have done. But Jack was different. Even though he was hearing, he was sensitive to my needs. He made me laugh and feel good about myself, like I had a lot to offer."

"Apparently including an ability to intuit his needs more than even he could!" I said.

Sheila blushed and said, "Well, yeah, I've always had a gift of being intuitive. After becoming deaf, I learned to read peoples' expressions pretty well. And Jack and I were quick soul mates. We could practically read each other's minds!"

"I'm intrigued though by your reference, 'he made me feel good about myself, like I had a lot to offer.' Would you tell us more about the part of you that may *not* have felt good about yourself or about what you had to offer?"

"Well, you know, many hearing people look at me like I'm deaf and dumb."

"Yeah, but that's what those hearing people may think. What about what you thought about yourself?"

"I know I'm intelligent, but it's hard being put down all your life. The negativity kind of gets to you after a while." Sheila was describing internalized oppression, when one comes to believe the negative cultural stereotypes about oneself. I needed to validate the existence of such discrimination and oppression—to agree that it's not in her head—and then ferret out how her low self-esteem may have contributed to their marital difficulties.

"I agree that unfortunately deaf-bashing is alive and well in this bigoted world of ours. But you're also saying that you also sometimes bash yourself, right?"

"Yeah, something like that" she replied. After a pause, she added, "My parents were thrilled that I married a hearing man."

"And why was that?"

"He could take care of me, be my 'ears to the world.'"

"Their message was that your deafness meant not being able to take care of yourself?"

"Right!" she replied.

"You know, we all begin long-term relationships with a list of 'thou shalts' and 'thou shalt nots,' what we want our partner to do and not to do. Our *conscious* expectations are easy. It's the unconscious ones that are tough."

Both Sheila and Jack nodded their heads, so I continued. "Sheila, it sounds like your initial, unspoken marital contract was that Jack would 'make' you feel better about yourself; and Jack, for you, it was that Sheila would 'make' your loneliness go away."

"We both failed miserably!" Sheila laughed. Jack also let out a wry laugh and nodded his head.

"Yeah, you blew it big time, but we all do. It always comes with long-term commitments. Painful as it may be, the initial breaching of our unconscious, implicit contracts is also a stepping stone to achieving deeper levels of intimacy and growth." They nodded their heads, either to be polite or to indicate tentative hope—I couldn't tell which.

We agreed to meet for weekly marital therapy with a general goal of "renegotiating their original, implicit marital contract." While writing my session notes, I thought of how, as with most couples, their implicit contract had worked fine for the first year or so: Jack was not lonely and Sheila liked herself more. However, they both ended up feeling let down by the other. A painful lesson: other people cannot take away our childhood pain.

During our next meeting, I asked them for some specifics to help fill in some gaps in their story. Married for 12 years, things had begun to go sour sometime after Sheila became pregnant with their son. In Sheila's words, "That's when I realized that Jack and I would be connected forever." A common sentiment but with an additional twist. She was conflicted about her hopes for her unborn child. Part of her wanted a child who was "deaf like me"—someone who would understand how it felt to be deaf in a hearing world—but she also "didn't want to inflict deafness on anyone."

Jack, however, was not conflicted at all. He had an irrational fear that his child would be born deaf.[a] He prayed every night that his children would be "normal," that they be spared the pain of a cruel, insensitive world that he had witnessed so many times through Sheila. But he felt he couldn't tell her about his fears, as it would "hurt her self-esteem even more." So he remained silent.

As it turned out, their child, named Stan, was hearing. His entrance into the world brought Sheila and Jack more immediate stress than joy: he had severe colic, seldom slept and, in their words, "wasn't the bundle of joy that we expected." In fact, his birth was the catalyst for Sheila making the appointment with me. Although she, in her words, "begged Jack for years to come with her to couples counseling," he finally acquiesced only when she threatened to sleep in a separate room with the baby. Jack would then be left alone.

It was time to explore how each of them enthusiastically, although unconsciously, accepted the terms of their original implicit marital

---

a. Sheila's deafness was not genetic or congenital and not likely to be genetically transmitted.

contract: how Jack accepted the role of filling up Sheila's self-esteem hole and how Sheila accepted the role of filling up Jack's loneliness hole. I asked Jack how he had first helped Sheila feel better about herself.

"Well, when we had people over for dinner, when we'd go to parties or church—when we were with almost any group of people—I would interpret by mouthing peoples' words. I'd tell her what was going on, what people were talking about. It was a lot of work!"

"Of course it was," I agreed. "But did this work also fulfill a need of yours?"

"Maybe you could say that."

"Go on," I smiled. He would have to do better than that.

"Well, it obviously felt good to be needed."

"What about feeling needed felt particularly good to you?" I asked.

"That she would always be there."

"'If Sheila is really dependent on me, she'll never leave?'" I asked.

"Maybe, but I didn't consciously think that! The way you put it sounds like leverage in a business deal." Jack became a bit defensive.

"Right. This is unconscious stuff," I said. "But there is some built-in power or leverage that hearing spouses have. We're given a lot of power in this hearing world of ours. In Sheila's parents' words, you became her 'ears to the world.'"

"I did depend on him a lot," Sheila jumped in.

"And how do you think Jack felt about himself when he became your ears?"

"I think it gave him a purpose. I think it felt good to him to be needed by me."

"What do you think, Jack?"

"There's some truth to that, I'll admit. It does feel good to be needed."

Sheila and Jack's situation illustrated a common cross-cultural exchange between Deaf and hearing persons. Although power and dependency must be negotiated as part of any relationship, they are more salient between these two cultures.[3] In an academic main-streaming situation, for example, a hearing student and a Deaf student may become friends. Although, for the most part, they may develop a reciprocal relationship, the Deaf peer obtains in the hearing friend both an interpreter (either oral or sign language) and a friend. The hearing peer is in a position to control much of the language and the information flow between the Deaf peer and the hearing group. The Deaf peer's dependency and the hearing peer's power threaten to pollute the friend part of the exchange.

Moreover, when the peer group attempts to converse with the Deaf person, the actual conversation will often be directed to the hearing peer: "Tell him...." The challenge is to work out a mutually empowering way of handling such omnipresent temptations toward imbalances of power. Easier said than done.

"And Sheila, how about you? How did you try to make Jack feel less lonely?"

She paused and her face blushed a bit. "Well, back then we had great sex!"

"Your ability to tune into his feelings helped connect both of you sexually?"

"Yeah, we both agreed that our sex was the best we've ever had with anyone! But it wasn't only that. I also became his confidant; he shared his deepest wishes and fears with me. He would always tell me that I could 'hear' him better than his hearing friends could."

"So you felt very special to him. Like you had the power to help him recognize and explore some deeply personal feelings?"

"Absolutely. That's why I didn't feel so bad when he would kind of interpret for me with other people, as his lips are easier to read. I knew I was giving him something back that no one else had ever given him before."

"And when did that feeling change for you?"

"After the birth of Stan."

"And why do you think that was?"

"Well, for one thing, Stan took up all of my time and energy."

"A very special bond happens between a mother and her baby. Many of us men envy it," I said, anticipating what was to come.

"Jack didn't say so at first, but I knew he was jealous. And love-making for the first several months? Ugh! It was the last thing I wanted!"

"We haven't made love in over a year," Jack scoffed. "*Now,* what's your excuse?"

"Lovemaking is a typical indicator of relationship difficulties," I quickly interjected. "I don't think we're ready to discuss this now. My suggestion is that we table this topic until later." It was too early in our relationship to get into that undoubtedly sensitive area, and it was a distraction from our needing to first understand the context in which lovemaking, or rather the lack thereof, was embedded.

As Jack nodded his head, I continued my discussion with Sheila: "So although a big part of your original implicit contract was to keep Jack from experiencing marital loneliness, that's precisely what happened with the birth of Stan?"

Both of them nodded their heads.

"Jack, would you put words to your nod? What are you thinking?" I asked.

"It sounds crazy, I know. But I was a bit jealous." After a pause, he continued: "Sheila used to kiss me goodbye every morning before work. But, after Stan was born, she said she needed more sleep; she told me not to wake her up in the morning; not to bother her; and to 'Be quiet when you get dressed.' It's almost like she couldn't wait to have me out of the house. I felt like—"

Now Sheila lunged forward in her seat. "Did you offer to take care of Stan in the middle of the night when he cried? Did you offer to change his diapers? Did you offer to burp him and give him his formula? Did you? Did you?" Sheila and Jack both knew the answer.

"Sheila, how did you feel when Jack didn't help you with all these things?"

"Pissed off! It was his sperm, too!"

"No one would argue with that," I smiled. Sheila did not return the smile, as she was understandably enraged. But her justified anger was not the full story. I had a sense that some additional pain, perhaps part of the reasons for her feelings of low self-esteem, was re-stimulated.

"Did you feel overwhelmed?" I asked.

"Big time! I had no fucking idea what to do with this baby who wouldn't stop crying, never slept, and always looked unhappy."

"And did Stan being hearing increase or decrease your feeling overwhelmed?"

"I don't know. Although I expected to have a hearing baby, it would have felt more familiar to me if he were Deaf."

"I see. And what did you say to yourself about yourself as you felt so overwhelmed?"

"I felt like the worst mother on this planet. I felt super inept."

"And where does that 'super inept' feeling bring you back to?"

Sheila thought for only a few seconds. She had taken this trip back many times before: "To feeling incompetent and left out when all the hearing people are talking around me..."

"On the one hand, your feelings of ineptness were what Jack was supposed to protect you from, just as you were supposed to protect him from his loneliness. On the other hand, both of you—like anyone in marriage—can grow precisely from reexperiencing the roots of your feelings of ineptness and loneliness with each other."

Jack and Sheila's so-called "breach of contract" echoed a profound duality inherent in most, if not all, committed relationships: that we are drawn to partners who will aid us in our search for wholeness, yet we run away at critical times in anger and fear. Ironically, we retreat precisely when the deepening intimacy of our relationships finally enables us to reclaim those essential, forgotten parts of ourselves. As author John Welwood noted, "Even couples who share a vision of their relationship as an opportunity for personal or spiritual development often find it hard to regard the difficulties in their way as creative challenges rather than intractable problems."[4]

"C'mon Mike," Jack scowled impatiently. "You mean if my dad

abused me, I should marry an abusive wife so I can reexperience the abuse and 'grow'?"

Sheila nodded her head. Interestingly, this was the first time I had seen them empathetically connect, but now against their therapist! As we were already ten minutes past the end of our meeting, I needed to wrap up our dialogue, hopefully in a way that would feel supportive.

"No, of course it's not that simple," I admitted, "and we need to stop for now. But, as a preview of some possible upcoming discussions, let me say this: that you may end up—to use your analogy— reexperiencing your wife as abusive *whether she is or not.* There's a bunch of theories why that happens, but I can assure you it's common. And I can also assure you—and maybe you have to take this on faith for the time being—that, if instead of running away from each other, you can learn to stay with your feelings, process them both internally and with each other, you'll reap many rewards."

Although Jack's conscious hope was for Sheila to somehow take away his loneliness, I believe that, at another less conscious level, he knew he needed to reexperience his loneliness with her in order to gain mastery over it. Similarly, I believed that, although Sheila's conscious hope was for Jack to somehow take away her low self-esteem, she, too, unconsciously, realized that she would heal emotionally only after first reexperiencing it with him.

The meeting had covered a lot of ground. They reported that much of it seemed clear to them, although they seemed confused at certain points. I was satisfied to leave some of our discussion unclear. Unconscious dynamics are anything but clear; and there is a great danger of overintellectualizing and preventing any real emotional growth. Their curiosity would hopefully provide an impetus for further visits, for doing the reparative and transformative work of exploring the source of their pain.

As Jack had an extended out-of-town business convention, we scheduled our fourth appointment in two weeks. We agreed to then chart a course of action, including deciding on the frequency of our meetings and a more specific formulation of our goals.

I found myself looking forward to our next session. Admittedly, I need to work harder at this with some people: fatigue and insecurity about doing a good enough job and intrusions from my personal life are all well-known culprits that get in my way. But I felt good about my beginning relationship with Jack and Sheila. I felt proud of them and of me for our brief but intense and productive contact.

It therefore came as a real surprise and a disappointment that they did not show for their next appointment. That night, Jack left a message on my answering machine thanking me for my time but saying that they decided not to "pursue couples counseling right now." A couple of days later, I got a similar note from Sheila.

Now I found myself doing a psychology "autopsy" of our meetings. What did I miss? What did I do wrong? Did we go too fast? Too slow? Did their conflicts escalate too intensely? Many unanswered questions. After several frustrating moments of head scratching, I had to let it go. There was food shopping to be done (my wife and I were having company that night), I needed to get gas, and my kids had to be picked up at soccer practice. In this case, these life distractions were welcome ones.

It was a year later, almost to the day, when I received a phone call from Jack. This time, it was *he* who requested an appointment. Two days later, Jack and Sheila entered my office and took the same seats as they had before. After exchanging pleasantries, I focused on a point between them and simply asked, "Who wants to start?"

Jack shifted uncomfortably in his seat. Sheila gave the command "Go on!" Her wrath was loud and clear.

After several more hesitations and awkward shifting, Jack took the plunge. He disclosed that he had been having an affair for over 13 months! At first it began innocently. An office party, lingering around for a drink or two, then casual banter and office gossip. He recalled thinking that it was a good way to let off stress and improve job performance. His rationalizations even included thinking that he could deduct all these costs as business-related expenses.

"The sequence is so obvious in retrospect," Jack lamented.

"It always is," I nodded my head. I shouldn't have been so stunned but I was. For me, too, it now seemed obvious in retrospect. When Sheila had originally "dragged him in to couples counseling," he was already in the early stages of an affair.

"An affair is a complicated thing," I said somewhat tentatively. "Let's try to at least begin to understand how and why it happened, and decide where you two want to go from here." I was unclear exactly why they were back. Did they want to pick up the pieces or get a divorce?

Jack recounted how clear it had all seemed. Monica was the woman that Sheila could never be: "She had a beautiful soul, she was sensitive, loving, giving..." Before I could interject, Jack said it for me: "I know what you're going to say: like I viewed Sheila when we first met."

I nodded my head.

"Sheila found out about her a month ago. But I was going to break it off anyway."

"How come?"

"A lot of reasons: guilt, feeling shitty about myself, and it turned out that Monica was no match to Sheila. I never appreciated what I already had." He began to sob. Sheila, however, remained stoic.

"What do you make of how it turned out?" I asked. "Did Monica change or did you?"

"Maybe a little bit of both."

"How so?" I prodded.

"Well, after a while, I took off my rose-colored glasses; and, after a while, she let her hair down."

"You saw her humanness."

"Yeah," Jack admitted sadly. "It's almost like being drunk," he said.

"I agree. Beginning romance is a kind of drunkenness. You can't see your partner clearly—whether it be a Sheila or a Monica or anyone else. Instead, you see them as goddesses. And they, too, show you only their best, 'rose-colored' side, saving their dark, more intimate side for later."

As the story unfolded, Jack recalled how he was so immersed in feelings of disconnection from Sheila that he could not imagine that she noticed the clues which in retrospect seemed absurdly obvious: the late nights at work, excessive care to his dress, increased exercise. Jack recalled feeling "a kind of magic, pure happiness and joy!"

"Like everything was different: people you disliked seemed nicer—"

"Yeah," he replied: "Colors were brighter, food tasted better, et cetera, et cetera." We both recalled him using almost the exact same words to describe his falling in love with Sheila.

People may react in a variety of ways when feeling betrayed and abandoned by their partners. Some get outright angry and even abusive. Others engage in addictive behaviors with alcohol, drugs, or food. Others become workaholics. Still others have affairs. All of these behaviors are designed to shield us from our pain. However, these avoidance strategies have a longer term opposite effect. Although they give us the illusion of fulfillment, in fact, they keep our painful emotions alive, festering just below the surface. That lesson was what Jack was only beginning to learn. Unfortunately, Sheila had been victimized in the process.

It was past time to acknowledge her victimization. "Sheila, to say the obvious, this has to be absolutely devastating to you."

Her face showed raw pain. There are few marital betrayals that are more common but more devastating. My heart went out to her.

"I can't tell you what this has done to me," she began. "For weeks, my stomach was in knots and I couldn't eat. I couldn't sleep. And I alternated between crying out of control and wanting to kill him. Every day, I kept looking at myself in the mirror, asking 'What's wrong with me? Why did he do this?'" Her eyes welled up.

"It wasn't you, Sheila. There's nothing wrong with you. I love you the way you are," Jack interjected in a desperate but futile attempt to be comforting.

"Shut up you son of a bitch," Sheila screamed.

For several moments we sat in silence. It was time to end. Who would have thought that this meeting—the one that was supposed to have happened a year ago when I was proud of our good work and confident of more to follow—would have come to this? As I sat with my own disappointment, this time it was me who felt betrayed, lied to by that "son of a bitch." Could they sense my disappointment and anger? Probably, was my inner answer. After another few seconds of silence and a deep breath, I chanted to myself, "let it go, let it go." I realized that we needed to acknowledge their crisis with as much neutrality as possible: it is a process, a journey, an adventure. I thought of Jerry Garcia's wisdom, "What a long, strange trip it's been." A common hearing-based behavior to associate life's moments with song lyrics.

I asked each of them to focus on their breathing, to acknowledge that they were each in crisis, albeit from very different positions, and also to acknowledge that they took a brave step in reopening a dialogue here.

Both of them requested another appointment to discuss "where we go from here." I readily agreed. But this time I knew better than to anticipate the next step. It is a lesson I keep relearning. Adventures are by definition unpredictable. Long, strange trips.

During the next week, I spent time thinking about the psychology of affairs and intimacy. Affairs are bounded by *space and time.* They occur in discrete environments—hotel rooms, out-of-the-way places—that are conducive to privacy and secrecy. And the rendezvous typically has a defined beginning and end, i.e., several hours, one evening, an out-of-town trip or over several months. It is the spatial and temporal *boundedness* of affairs that gives them their bursting flame, high intensity. But its intensity is often confused with intimacy. In fact, affairs are *pseudo*intimate encounters, precisely because they are so bounded.

In contrast, long-term, committed relationships lack the fireworks intensity of affairs, but contain precious growth opportunities

that come from working through crises (conflict, loss, etc.) and dealing with unstructured "down time." With these challenges, however,
also come anxiety and fear. I am reminded of two friends who took
a long car trip together. One of them began an intimate, deep topic
with the other only when both knew that there was only one-half
hour left.

I wondered what the next part of Sheila and Jack's adventure
would be.

Sheila wasted no time in beginning our next meeting. She announced that she had told Jack to move out. It would be a trial separation for an indefinite period, a time, in her words, "for me to
heal." Stan would remain with her. Jack would have liberal visitation
rights.

Jack's response to this news was solemn and repentant. It had obviously not come as a complete surprise. Several times he said, "I'll
do whatever you need."

"Could you talk more about what you need to heal?" I asked
Sheila.

Her response was reminiscent of other spouses who learn of their
partner's infidelity. "I find myself wanting but not wanting to know
all the details. What she did for him, how they made love, when he
lied to me, whether he thought about her when *we* made love, what
he bought her, what she gave him. And since I'm deaf I don't hear
what he says on the phone. Did he phone her from our house?" She
had endless questions.

Sheila brought to mind one more question of my own: "Have you
been curious about whether Monica is hearing or Deaf?"

"I already know that she's hearing," came her quick response. "He
leaves me with the kid and gets his rocks off with a real, hearing
woman!"

"What he did must play into your worst fears about being with a
hearing man: that he would demean you in some way. Reinforce
that hearing is real; deafness is unreal."

"Yeah, I've thought of that. Him cheating on me is my worst

nightmare." For an instant it looked like she would cry, but then, as if to deny him the power of seeing her so vulnerable, she clenched her fists instead.

On a universal level, "cheating" would be any spouse's worst nightmare. However, with Jack and Sheila in particular, there was a unique repercussion having to do with oppressed minority group dynamics. Consider an interracial couple in which the wife is Black and the husband is White. If the White husband has an affair with a woman who is also White, he could inflict a wound on his Black wife that could echo years of cultural degradation that White people are better than Black people. The sentiment that "hearing is real, deafness is unreal" was reminiscent of how oppressed minorities are dehumanized—made unreal.

With Sheila, it would be important to help her give the feelings generated by her "worst nightmare" a voice, both with herself during private moments of reflection and with Jack. We discussed at length that this process would be excruciatingly painful, and that, in large part, it would entail her grieving a major loss, in this case the marital trust and security that she had taken for granted. I explained to her that, contrary to popular belief, one does not master the stages of grieving in a finite time period and arrive at acceptance. However, having seen this process many times before, I assured her that she would not only get through it, but that there would be personal rewards along the way. In response to her shaking her head in disbelief, I asked her to at least know that I believed my prediction. She nodded her head.

Jack and Sheila were beginning a long journey of discovery and healing. It was a beginning because Jack had been having an affair when we had first met and had little or no interest in working on his marriage or himself. Now at least both of them were engaged in an honest dialogue and effort. The three of us agreed on weekly meetings as an integral part of their emotional work during their separation. (He found an apartment a few miles away). They also agreed to go out together as a couple at least once weekly—not to have a good time as if nothing had happened, but rather to ensure ongoing space and time for their dialogue and exploration. In addition, at my recommendation, both of them agreed to begin individual therapy to work on personal issues.

It would have been a mistake to encourage them to forego any contact with each other and have individual therapy in order to "find out who you really are." It does not work that way. Retreat does not lead to true individuation. Rather, we individuate—develop a mature sense of who we are—as a result of forging out our needs and wants from those of our partners through clarification, assertiveness, and compromise. Individuation is not a by-product of only our own "hero's journey," nor of only the good times of relationships. It is also very much a by-product of the interplay of lightness and darkness inherent in every long-term, committed relationship.

I was reminded of a story told by a Jungian analyst, Jean Shinoda Bolen. She once led a group of women into an underground cavern where they were told to sit still for hours without light or discussion. Upon returning to the light, nobody reported enjoying the experience of darkness, but everybody said they benefited from it. The group coined the term "endarkenment" to describe the archetypal wisdom that comes with going into the darkness and coming back again.

My task was to help Sheila and Jack to tolerate and explore their darkness, the disowned, split-off parts of their consciousness that became visible only *as a result of* their relationship struggles. For Sheila, her cavern contained the belief that deafness meant inferiority: the medical model of deafness. Sheila reported that she would work on finding her own voice, her own power, and on not letting others—i.e., her mother, husband, boss, the hearing culture—steal it from her. Jack's cavern contained the belief that he was not a worthwhile person unless he took care of others in a more or less codependent manner. Moreover, he also suffered from a fragile self-esteem. He planned to work on developing his ability to enjoy being with himself when he was alone, rather than retreat, feel abandoned, and/or have affairs.

We also had a lot of cleanup to do from Jack's affair. In reaction to hearing Sheila's anger and pain, Jack would typically feel guilty and then immediately retreat or say a platitude like "it's behind us, let's move on." I repeatedly explained to him that moving on too quickly was wishful thinking. In addition to grief and recovery work, Sheila needed to understand the reasons for his affair as reflecting Jack's fears and anxieties about what got stirred in him by their marriage, rather than attributing his affair to deficits with her.

While living separately, they journeyed into their respective dark caverns through their own personal therapeutic work, couples meetings, and regular interchanges with each other, both in my office and out in the "real world," as they put it. And in six months, they came to a critical juncture: one that all successful couples typically look back on as the turning point in their marriages. Jack and Sheila came to experience themselves as strong enough, stable enough, and able enough to actively *make a choice* about the future of their relationship. Each of them could decide to go either way: remain married or be divorced. It was no longer a given that they *had to* remain entangled in matrimony; each could survive financially, each would likely meet another partner, each would live a happy and productive life, their child would do fine and it did not matter what the relatives would think. Their personal liberation was in marked contrast to earlier feelings of entrapment, "being stuck with each other," having only a choiceless choice of whether to stay married.

One day they began their meeting with "cautious optimism." Sheila announced that she had asked Jack to move home that weekend.

"Why now?" I asked.

Jack responded with, "What happened was—"

"He asked me," Sheila interrupted.

I smiled and Jack smiled, too.

"Go on, please," I beckoned her.

"I've forgiven Jack although there are periods—and probably always will be—that I think of Monica and want to cry or scream. But these times are fleeting and they don't consume me like they used to. And—not that I would wish what happened to me on my worst enemy—my reconciling Jack's affair made me realize that I'm a good, attractive, worthwhile partner. Now, the work that we have to do on our relationship can only be done living together." Sheila then elucidated some of what she termed the "day-to-day challenges" of maintaining her sense of self in the context of an intimate relationship, "balancing the I and we."

Sheila emerged from her metaphorical cavern with newfound strength or endarkenment. She proved to herself that she did not need a man (one day she came in wearing a shirt that said A Woman Needs a Man Like a Fish Needs a Bicycle). Even more importantly, Sheila proved to herself that she did not need a *hearing* man to be, as her parents would say, her "ears to the world" or a "human hearing aid." She told Jack and me that if her parents were to say again that "Your hearing husband can take care of you," she would give them a well-rehearsed reply:

> Mom, Dad, I love Jack for many reasons, but they don't include him having brown hair, blue eyes or working ears. These are all superficial qualities. I'm proud of him and I'm proud of me for doing some hard work on our marriage and ourselves. I very much need the love and intimacy that we have achieved. But I don't need him to take care of me; and I certainly don't need his ears.

Jack emerged from his cave learning to tolerate the parts of himself that he had not dared explore before: his emptiness, loneliness, and vulnerability—pain that came from his childhood, largely spent disconnected from his parents. Like many of us, he had previously discounted the present effects of the distant past, with the saying "today is the first day of the rest of my life." He learned an essential paradox: *you can be liberated from the past only when you can accept that it is always there.* Now Jack no longer had to distract himself from his inner cave by being Sheila's "ears to the world" or by having affairs. He no longer had to psychologically self-medicate his emptiness away.

The three of us continue to meet, on a weekly or biweekly basis. At this writing, we have met about 50 times. The issue of trust occupies much of our time, as Sheila begins to develop more confidence in Jack's fidelity, while Jack does his own essential work. Among other standard challenges that all couples face, they are also working hard to negotiate those that are unique to hearing-deaf couples: i.e., when/how/if Jack interprets social conversation for Sheila and vice versa, when/how/if Sheila says to Jack that she does not want to go to hearing social functions and vice versa. All in all, they are doing well.

When I think of Jack and Sheila, I marvel at the reparative power of committed love. Through their marriage, Sheila reclaimed her lost competence and Jack reclaimed more emotional self-sufficiency. How do our partners aid us in our search for wholeness? From stories such as Jack and Sheila's, it seems to me that committed partners provide us with a safe place where we can reexperience and therefore recover our childhood joys as well as reexperience and therefore master our previous wounds and the foundations of our inner caves. There is an extraordinary transformative power that comes with having the guts to continually work at integrating the lightness and darkness of our committed relationships. They are indeed "long, strange trips."

Notes

1. Hendrix, H. (1988). *Getting the love you want: A guide for couples.* New York: HarperPerennial.

2. Hendrix, H. (1988). *Getting the love you want: A guide for couples.* New York: HarperPerennial.

3. Hoffmeister, R., & Harvey, M. A. (1998). "Is there a psychology of the hearing?" In N.S. Glickman & M.A. Harvey (eds.). *Culturally affirmative psychotherapy with Deaf persons.* Mahwah, NJ: Lawrence Erlbaum.

4. Welwood, J. (1997). *Love and awakening: Discovering the sacred path of intimate relationship.* New York: HarperPerennial.

CHAPTER 3

Demilitarizing the Parent-Teacher Battle Zone

Paul, a 15-year-old, hard-of-hearing adolescent, appeared at my office. Usually parents don't have to bribe their children to get them to agree to see a therapist. But Paul could be quite stubborn. So they promised him new computer video software after each visit. Not a bad deal.

I imagined that he had to work especially hard to appear so slovenly for our initial meeting: his hair was filthy and greasy, his pants were torn and oil stained, his t-shirt depicted blood and gore, and he emitted a repugnant cigarette odor. He did not speak, but his nonverbal communications were clear.

Although he walked into my office on his own accord, I imagined his parents leveling the equivalent to a powerful shove on his behind in addition to visits to the software store. He plopped on the chair closest to the door and gave me a passive, hostile stare.

I attempted to establish rapport: "Nice shirt! How ya doin? How's school? How's home? What do you do for fun with your friends?"

Paul was the only child of two hearing parents, Shawn and Margaret Smith, and had incurred a moderate hearing loss soon after his second birthday, cause unknown. Although he was fitted with two hearing aids, he said his hearing loss was "no big deal." Half of the time at school, he would forget to wear his aids. He had excellent oral/aural skills and appeared to speech read me well. At least in my quiet, well-lit office, our linguistic communication would not be the problem.

My first task was to clarify my role. I gave Paul my usual speech that my job was to "advise your parents what they can do to help you," "talk about emotional stuff," "help you be happier," etc. I ended with "seeing a psychologist doesn't mean you're crazy." He nodded his head.

My second task was to ask if he knew why he was here. He replied, "I don't know."

But his parents knew. Whereas Shawn confided in me that he agreed to outside-of-school psychotherapy only to get the school off his back, Margaret reported that she had always been concerned about Paul's oppositional behavior at home and school. She vacillated between blaming the school, her husband, herself, and Paul. Now she was leaning toward holding the school accountable. She wanted my input.

Paul, however, was not about to talk about emotional issues. Our discussion was limited to comparing the pros and cons of different computer games and "how boring school is." When I asked him why school was so boring, he replied, "I don't know; it just is." If I had a nickel for how many times adolescents say "I don't know" or "boring," I would be a rich man. Paul was no exception.

After almost an hour had elapsed, he displayed another version of his passive-aggressive stance. He looked at me with mock befuddlement and asked, "Isn't it time to stop now?"

I replied, "I don't know." For the first time, he couldn't help but smile. We made tentative eye contact. I shook his hand and said that I'd be in touch.

On paper, his academic placement looked good. Although he was the only hearing-impaired student in a huge mainstream environment, his individualized educational plan specified the full-time services of an oral interpreter, an FM system, preferential seating and a host of other accommodations. However, contrary to Paul's self-report, the school indicated that he not only struggled to understand the formal instruction of many of his teachers, but also resigned himself to missing most of the social chit-chat, incidental information, and social cues from other students. Apparently, the design of the classroom was an acoustic nightmare.

Behaviorally, he was a terror. Paul frequently disrupted the classroom, was rude to teachers and other students, refused to follow instructions, and had poor impulse control and a short attention span. He didn't get along with his peers and often started fights that he always deemed "someone else's fault." As a result of the psychologist stating in his report that Paul had attention deficit disorder (ADD) and telling the teachers, off the record, that "he has pent up rage toward his parents that gets displaced onto other authority figures," the school set up a structured behavior program for Paul at lightning speed.

Although the written psychological findings and recommendations in the official report sparked marked relief from Paul's teachers, they sparked anger from his parents. They had accumulated an impressive casebook of documented, dated allegations against the school for having caused most, if not all, of Paul's problems: when "Paul's teacher bawled him out and embarrassed him in front of the whole class," "when the teachers didn't give him enough visual cueing," "when they misunderstood certain nuances of his speech," "when they put mean ideas about the family into his head," "when they didn't call us," etc. Their closing argument was *the mainstream teaching staff doesn't understand about hearing loss and lacks sensitivity.*

However, the teachers also took the role of plaintiff. They resented Paul's parents for what they perceived as their "emotional neglect," "intrusiveness in the classroom," and "offensive insinuations." They, too, had amassed an impressive array of incriminating documentation, which included "when mother came in the classroom unannounced and caused disruption by her relentless questioning," "when they seemed so disinterested and bothered by us," and "when mother inappropriately yelled at Paul during a school meeting." The teachers also noted that his parents "didn't even have a TV decoder at home," "don't set enough limits" and "often send him to school without his hearing aids." The teachers' closing argument: *"Paul's parents don't understand about hearing loss and lack sensitivity."*

Paul, however, was not an innocent bystander to this escalating conflict around him. In fact, he expertly played one side against the other, a skill that he had slowly and carefully mastered as a child by playing Mom against Dad. Paul articulately complained to his teachers that his parents were grossly unfair and he articulately complained to his parents that his teachers were grossly unfair. He portrayed himself as the victim to both parties.

A predictable but unfortunate scenario: When the teachers had followed the recommendations of the report by setting up a well-designed behavior modification program for Paul, it was doomed to failure. When he suffered negative consequences at school for his poor classroom behavior, he was comforted by his parents upon returning home, as they pitied him for having been mistreated. In this manner, his parents colluded with Paul against the school.

At the same time, the teachers at school, in frustration over attempting to manage Paul's behavior and not obtaining parental cooperation, found themselves alternately acting excessively harshly toward Paul or giving up and excusing his inappropriate behavior. Occasionally, some teachers even expressed sympathy directly to Paul when he tearfully exaggerated his maltreatment at home. In this manner, the teachers colluded with Paul against his parents whom they accused of "undoing what we're trying to do at school."

From each side, he received sympathy and at least tacit support. Progress at school was undone at home; and progress at home was undone at school.

It would have been simple to diagnose Paul as having *the problem* and to provide individual treatment accordingly. The psychological evaluation had documented that he had ADD; his parents and teachers had reported that he was frequently oppositional; and his appearance in my waiting room had earned second glances from even those adolescents who also prided themselves on making a statement by their dress.

Individual diagnoses have the advantage of clarity. Moreover, with the DSM IV,[a] you can even assign five-digit numbers for any condition; in Paul's case, 313.81 for oppositional disorder and 314.01 for attention deficit hyperactivity disorder. A neat package. In contrast, the myriad, multilevel interactions within Paul's family, within the school system, and between the school and parents were not simple.

From my experience, it is common for deaf or hard-of-hearing students to display behavioral problems in school as a reaction to discord between their teachers and parents. The reasons for this situation are complex. Both parents and teachers may view the student's behavior as reflective of their own competency. Parents of disabled children, in particular, may have a heightened sensitivity to potentially negative external influences—e.g., teachers "who don't understand him/her like we do." As a parent of a hard-of-hearing child said, "I can't let Johnny suffer any more from incompetent teachers than he already has because of his hearing loss."

Similarly, teachers who have a deaf/hard-of-hearing student(s) in their classroom may find themselves colluding with the student against his/her parents. Some teachers deem the parents as not motivated enough to "make the child as hearing as possible." Certified teachers of the Deaf often find themselves trying to undo the communication inaccessibility of the student's home environment. As one teacher said, "I sign much better than those parents do."

My position with respect to the adversarial parties around Paul was crucial. First I needed to ensure a strong alliance with all parties,

---

a. *The Diagnostic and Statistical Manual,* 4th edition (DSM IV), is the official listing of psychiatric diagnoses, published by the American Psychiatric Association.

particularly Paul's parents whom I had just met. Then I would become a diplomat of sorts between the school and parents. Finally, I would invite Paul to witness first-hand the demilitarized parent-teacher battle zone and thus be disentangled—"detriangulated"—from their conflict. The plan of action: (1) family meeting(s); (2) a meeting(s) with Paul's parents and selected school personnel; (3) a meeting(s) with Paul, his parents, and teachers together; and (4) a listing of some of my own recommendations.

At the family meeting a week later, Paul and his parents presented themselves as a cohesive army combat unit. Whereas they had often fought with each other about Paul cleaning up his room, combing his hair, keeping curfew, his attitude, etc., now all three family members were solidly united against the big, bad school. A common enemy stabilizes even the most precarious relationships. My attempts to redirect them to look at their own difficulties and conflicts proved futile. Instead, they came back with more accusations against the school, inevitably followed by "Dr. Harvey, what do you think?"

Some of their complaints, however, seemed valid. The teachers had never received in-service training on hearing loss issues and the acoustics in the classroom were horrendous. However, as with most adversarial situations, their perceptions of the other tended to be distorted *half*-truths. And they steadfastly insisted on viewing the school as having started any and all conflicts. "They're incompetent; they should all be fired!" came their battle cries. I had unwelcome flashbacks to the hopeless quagmire of trying to figure out which one of my kids "started" a particular fight: "But, Daddy, Alli did.... But, Daddy, Emily did..."

I did my best to duck the family's attempts to get me to collude with them against the school. Instead, I conveyed sympathy for them having such an antagonistic relationship and repeatedly wondered how it may be affecting Paul's behavior, both at school and at home. At this point in our discussion, Paul began to shift uncomfortably in his seat.

Surprisingly, his parents immediately gave an accurate and succinct response: "He gets away with murder!"

"Tell me more." I said. Maybe their wrath at the school hadn't completely distracted them from acknowledging Paul's difficulties.

"You know," Shawn began, "he's not doing his homework, he talks back all the time, doesn't help with the..."

"But you're never home! How do you know?" Margaret interrupted.

"I know what I see when..." Shawn responded, now getting angry.

Paul's fidgetiness now dramatically decreased. When his parents began to fight with each other, he was no longer in the hot seat.

My turn to interrupt: "Whoa, hold on. Remember what you said: 'He gets away with murder.' And that means that it doesn't matter who's right and who's wrong. Your son's the main casualty in this war. All of us—you, me, and the school—need to come up with a plan. It's time to have a summit conference."

"I'm just tired of my wife always—"

"Never mind that for now!" I said while making the sign for time-out. "Declare a truce. Otherwise, you may win the battle, but you'll lose the war."

Now they nodded their heads in tentative agreement and at least temporarily threw down their firearms. Paul began to fidget again.

An expected occurrence in family therapy: my more solid alliance with Shawn and Margaret threatened my alliance with Paul. He now looked at me maliciously and I imagined he was planning his next maneuver. But I couldn't help but smile to myself. It's initially tough for kids, but ultimately necessary and beneficial, when the warring adults around them finally declare a cease-fire and begin team-building. Hopefully, Paul would not raise the stakes by acting out more.

"Hey, Paul," I said, trying to win him over, "If your parents and teachers get their act together, what do you think would change for you?"

"I don't know," he said. Predictable.

"Well I know that it'll be good for Paul," Margaret emphatically said. Shawn nodded his head. But all Paul did was fidget more.

As we prepared to end our session, I joked that we should see how much it costs to rent Camp David, the setting where, in 1978, President Carter facilitated an accord between Egyptian President Anwar Sadat and Israeli Prime Minister Menachem Begin. However, Shawn had apparently returned to battle, as he sarcastically dismissed any possibility for an amicable accord with a sarcastic "yeah right!" He then suggested instead that "we may be able to catch them off guard if we meet on their turf." So much for the cease-fire. Paul, however, now looked noticeably more relaxed.

At the parents-school meeting one month later, we met in the school psychologist's office. In attendance were John, the school psychologist; Lauren, Paul's primary teacher; and his parents. The principal was "busy." Paul knew about our meeting but emphasized that, even if he were invited, he wouldn't want to come to anything "so boring."

As before, everyone was seated around a long conference table and appeared pleasant and amiable. They shared their hopes that others were "doing fine" and were sure to comment on what nice weather we'd been having.

I broke the small-talk (the tension was palpable) by asking that I be given the authority to regulate and interrupt the discussion if it strayed from our shared goals. At the outset, I wished to firmly establish my role as the leader with the means to bypass open warfare. A rigid structure would be critical, at least for now, much like the necessity of putting a cast around a broken bone. They unanimously agreed.

My next task was to acknowledge and begin diffusing the complex sequence of misunderstandings, disappointments, betrayals, and grievances that had preceded this meeting. I suggested that "it would be easy but unproductive to talk the past, as we would get lost in the chicken and egg cycle of who started it." I wanted to avoid what is called the "what happened" conversation and the "blame frame." Professors Stone, Patton and Heen, in their aptly titled book *Difficult Conversations,* point out that "difficult conversations are almost never about getting the facts right... and most focus significant attention on who's to blame for the mess we're in."[1]

While the three most important words in real estate are "location, location, and location," the three most important words in conflict resolution are "expectations, expectations, and expectations." But they have to be very specific and concrete. I made a strong pitch for us to focus on each person's expectations of each other from *that moment on.*

Everyone nodded their heads. One by one, the participants agreed that they wanted "increased cooperation," "better coordination," and "more support." Predictably, my task was to help operationalize these well-intentioned but much-too-vague goals.

"Let's make a list," I suggested. I also asked for a volunteer note taker. Lauren raised her hand.

Everybody wanted a coordinated way to monitor Paul's academic progress. Accordingly, I asked the teachers and parents to jointly design a weekly checklist system. (I thought of the social psychology experiment when two antagonist groups at a summer camp finally became friends when they had to cooperate in a joint venture in order to win a prize). After some initial awkwardness, they got to work. My role was to ensure that their hands-on joint venture stayed on track.

The target behaviors for school were Paul staying in his seat, watching the oral interpreter, wearing his hearing aids, and finishing tasks; and the target behaviors for home were Paul doing homework and bringing his books to school. On Fridays, he would ask his teachers to initial the list and then bring it home to his parents. We agreed that if Paul for whatever reason happened to "forget" the list—leaving it at school or at home, giving it to a dog, etc.—he would be required to *watch* his father play his favorite computer game all weekend but would be prohibited from playing it himself. Certain torture.

As the group finished their task, Margaret chimed in with "I just know he'll throw a temper tantrum!"

Shawn gave her a nasty look. Lauren gave Shawn a nasty look. A quick intervention: "Let's design a behavior plan to minimize Paul's temper tantrums," I suggested to Margaret and Shawn.

"Now?" they asked in unison.

"Yeah, let's spend some time—just the three of us while we give the school folks a break—figuring out a behavior plan you could use: some positive and negative consequences." I wanted to *exclude* the "school folks" from this process, as their participation would likely have been viewed by the parents as competitive. At first reluctantly, but then with more momentum, Shawn and Margaret forged out a plan with built-in positive reinforcements, logical consequences, etc. During this process, I noticed out of the corner of my eyes that the teachers looked pleased to see Shawn and Margaret invested in problem-solving and hard at work. The parents' devotion was not new; but it had been camouflaged by the layers of conflict and communication breakdowns.

Immediately after they finished, Margaret looked at Lauren and asserted that she expected better classroom management of Paul. Although the abruptness of her request suggested some defensiveness on her part for having been the object of focus, it was a reasonable request. Accordingly, I suggested to the school psychologist and teacher that they brainstorm about different classroom approaches while Margaret and Shawn observed. We discussed interventions for when Paul has difficulty sitting still or paying attention as well as when he becomes oppositional. Shawn and Margaret seemed pleased, now seeing more clearly the staff's devotion. That, too, had been camouflaged.

I continued asking each side what specific behaviors would constitute "support, cooperation, and coordination" from the other. Shawn requested that he would like the teacher to call him at work "if Paul has to be sent to the principal's office." Lauren agreed.

"Call you when?" I interrupted. "That very minute, hour, day, week, month?" Without adequate specificity, their well-intentioned goal was doomed to result in renewed warfare.

"Oh, I don't know," Margaret jumped in. "As soon as you can." Shawn looked displeased.

"Flexibility is fine," I quickly jumped in, "but not now. Let's not be too *falsely* nice. You guys are still cautiously looking each other over. It'll take time for trust to build up again. True flexibility comes only with trust. So, if for no other reason than just to humor me [now directly looking at Shawn], please specify *exactly* when you would like a phone call from Lauren." In addition to my prodding Shawn to be excruciatingly specific and deflecting his imminent attack on Margaret, I wanted to normalize present and future occurrences of tension between the school and parents.

Shawn said, "Before 3:00 that day."

"A.M. or P.M.?" I asked.

With tension-reducing laughter, Shawn replied, "In the afternoon would be fine."

"Good," I responded. "And what if you aren't available?"

"She can page me."

"Does she have your pager number?"

"Uh, no. Here it is." Shawn gave Lauren his pager number.

"Okay," I persisted. "But what about other less severe disciplinary actions that could be levied on Paul, ones that don't get him sent to the principal's office?" All parties then agreed that, in those cases, Lauren would fax Margaret a note describing the incident(s) sometime that day.

"So, [to Lauren] the request is for you to call Shawn before 3 P.M. that day if Paul has to be sent to the principal's office and if Shawn isn't available, to page him. For all lesser offenses, the request is for you to fax a brief note to Margaret anytime that day. Is this arrangement do-able?" I asked.

"Absolutely," Lauren said. She looked pleased, I imagined because the "broken bone" (their conflict) was finally put in a "cast" (clarification of specific expectations).

We were on a roll. The parents voiced their expectation for teachers to receive in-service training about hearing loss. They also wanted the opportunity to observe in the classroom. The teachers wanted adequate notice for parental visits, defined as at least 48 hours via a phone conversation with the respective teacher. They also requested that Paul's parents purchase a TV captioning device "to help him with his English." Onc by one, they reached agreement on these and other expectations.

Requests that the group could not reach agreement on—e.g., installing rugs and acoustic tiles in the classroom—were tabled until another meeting. First, as in the case of environmental modifications, some requests required outside administrative approval. Second, it would be important for them to forge a critical mass of agreements before tackling more difficult issues. They needed to have at least the beginnings of trust established.

I mentioned how much it touched me to see everyone's shared concern for Paul; the tension had been blocking it. Indeed everyone seemed more relaxed, as if they blew a collective sigh of relief. We would end the one-and-a-half-hour meeting on this positive note. However, it would have been a serious error to congratulate ourselves on a job well done and therefore expect that we would live "happily ever after," that there would not be renewed conflict. Change is neither easy nor quick. I emphasized to the group that "only on hour-long TV shows does one meeting cure everything."

"Not true with soap operas," Margaret noted.

Lauren laughed and said, "Yeah, they take all year!"

"Well, this group should take between one episode and one year," I laughed. "It's not *if* conflict happens, it's *when.* These struggles are part of all worthwhile relationships!" My intent was not to be pessimistic, but to provide a realistic and supportive framework that would destigmatize and normalize conflict and in which there was room for creative problem solving.

I also suggested that, due to the seriousness of Paul's behavior and to their tenuous, new-found alliance, Lauren and either Margaret or

Shawn should have daily phone contact for the next several weeks to "keep the lines of communication open." Everyone agreed. Finally, the school psychologist asked whether we would all want to meet again in a month, this time with Paul. There was unanimous and enthusiastic agreement. Margaret volunteered to bring donuts; the school would supply coffee for the adults and soda for Paul.

One month later, we assembled in the school psychologist's office, but this time, Paul and the principal were present (I think he showed up because he was curious what would happen). The "It's nice weather we're having, isn't it?" sugarcoated hostility was gone. Margaret was busy unpacking an assortment of donuts, Lauren and Shawn were pouring coffee, and John was putting out the cream and sugar. He wanted to know "Who took milk?" The principal handed Paul a can of ginger ale and asked him whether he wanted a straw. A now very stunned-looking boy replied "No, thank you."

"This is great coffee!" Shawn remarked. "What is it?"

"It's specialty coffee, hazelnut I think," Lauren proudly responded. Margaret asked where she could get some and said to her husband, "You never said that about *my* coffee!" Everyone laughed. "You never bought hazelnut before," he smiled. "How's your ginger ale?" the principal asked Paul. "Fine," he said.

After a bit more banter, we continued on to the formal agenda. First, a review of progress. Lauren and Margaret had daily phone contact for the first couple of weeks and then mutually agreed to decrease the frequency to weekly. Paul was sent to the principal's office twice, on which days Lauren phoned Shawn before 3:00 P.M. The checklist was going between home and school mostly without a hitch, except for once when Paul "forgot it." Accordingly, Shawn apparently had to play, in his words, "those damn computer games" while Paul watched. Finally, the school had scheduled an in-service training on hearing loss. They had asked Paul to participate but he had refused.

His behavior, however, had not improved; it had even gotten

worse. It was as if he were testing the limits. Sure enough, in the middle of the meeting, he complained to his mom that "the school was being too unfair."

Margaret responded with "Don't tell me, tell them! Then we can all talk about it!"

"What are we being unfair about?" John asked.

"I don't know, you just are."

"You need to tell them, son," Shawn said. "Otherwise, they won't know. Our job" he continued, motioning to every adult in the room, "is to help you live up to your potential. We're all committed to doing that here, because we all care about you."

Paul's attempts at igniting renewed conflict were fruitless. Instead, to his dismay and, I think, partial relief, his parents and teachers began to problem solve. Paul witnessed their effective teamwork from one end of what probably seemed like a very long table. Although he lost his means of colluding with one side against the other, he would get back the cohesive support and guidance of his parents and teachers.

My final intervention was the most straightforward: namely, my giving the school some specific recommendations. Over the years, I have created a list of common school-based interventions that may be helpful for hard-of-hearing students in mainstream settings, particularly for those students who demonstrate social and emotional difficulties. This listing has become a kind of boiler-plate from which I pick and modify the recommendations that apply to a specific student, such as Paul. The complete list is reprinted in an appendix following this chapter.[b]

Several months after the final hazelnut coffee and donut meeting, I received a call from Margaret. She happily reported that Paul had "finally come around" and improved his grades as well as his class-

---

b. My thanks to Marylyn Howe and Carol Menton for their contributions. I welcome suggestions from readers, as the listing is always being revised.

room behavior. The school had hired an audiologist to evaluate the acoustic environment and modifications were well underway. His behavior at home was "not perfect but much better."

"That's great to hear," I responded.

"But Shawn and I are having problems. He does... and doesn't..." she searched for the right words.

I laughed and asked, "And what do you think Shawn would say if I asked him?"

Now Margaret laughed: "Well, I guess he would probably complain that I do... and don't..."

"Where have we heard this before?" I laughed. No longer distracted by their conflict with Paul or with the school, Margaret and Shawn came face to face with their longstanding conflicts with each other. Per their request, we would meet later for marital therapy. But first, they wanted to have a family appointment with Paul "to reinforce his progress."

Several days later, we met. Both Shawn and Margaret were appropriately congratulatory of Paul for his improvement. Despite his attempts at sloughing off their complements, he looked pleased. Then came my natural question: "Why?"

The proud parents looked at their son. "Paul, why do think you're doing better?" Shawn asked.

Naturally, he gave his signature response. Accompanied by a well-rehearsed shrugging of his shoulders and furrowing of his eyebrows, he said *"I don't know."*

Appendix A

Common Recommendations for Hard-of-Hearing Mainstream Students Who Demonstrate Social/Emotional Difficulties

I.   Regarding the Student's Academic Functioning

- In-service training on issues relating to hearing impairment should be provided for all school personnel, including the substitute teacher(s) who may interact with the student. Such training should include sensitizing teachers to the often invisible effects of hearing loss. Appropriate cassette tapes for this purpose include Speech Through Amplification, available from the Speech and Hearing Clinic at University of Connecticut (860-486-3687), and Getting Through, available from Self Help for Hard of Hearing People (301-657-2248). In addition, all classroom teachers should be provided with a list of teaching hints for hard-of-hearing students.

- A program consultant regarding hearing loss should monitor the school program at least on an annual basis. The consultant's qualifications should preferably include a certificate of clinical competence in audiology, i.e., a CCC-A from ASHA.

- Note: The specifics of this recommendation should be confirmed by a qualified audiologist and may be modified accordingly.

   The school should make any necessary acoustical modifications to all rooms in which the student will receive academic instruction, e.g., mainstream classroom, resource room, speech therapy room and computer lab. It is my understanding from the acoustic environmental literature that two important factors are the *signal to noise ratio* and *reverberation.*

   The signal to noise ratio refers to the level of background noise that interferes with one's ability to understand speech. I believe that an acceptable standard is that the signal to noise ratio should be at least 20dB. This means that the teacher's voice would be at least 20dB louder than any background noise. However, this standard is variable, depending on the person's hearing acuity, audiometric configuration, etc.

Reverberation is the persistence of multiple reflections (or echoes) in an enclosed space. If there is insufficient sound-absorbing materials, such as tiles or carpets in the classroom or resource room or elsewhere, these reverberations will interfere with the hard-of-hearing person's understanding of speech.

I believe that a reverberation time of no greater than 0.5 seconds is an acceptable standard. However, in the student's case, this should be confirmed by an audiological engineer.

To reduce the reverberation and its concomitant interference with the signal to noise ratio, carpeting and acoustical ceiling tiles should be installed. Fluorescent lights and heating apparatus should be tested for excessive noise and should be repaired, if necessary. All rooms in which the student receives academic instruction should be located away from sources of externally generated noise, such as the gymnasium, shop, music room, cafeteria, and playground.

The implementation of this recommendation should be supervised by a qualified acoustic engineer and/or audiologist.

- Consultation from a certified and licensed audiologist is recommended concerning the advisability of the student using an FM transmitter/receiver or other assistive listening devices.

- The student's program should provide for hearing and hearing aid monitoring (audiological assessments to be performed at a local speech and hearing clinic, as needed). The school should identify staff who will monitor hearing and hearing aids during school hours and who are trained to troubleshoot minor problems, such as ear mold adjustment, tube replacement, and FM receiver modifications.

- All equipment (tape and record player, film projector, VCRs, etc.) should be checked for sound quality. All educational videos and television programming made available to other students should be made available to the student with captioning. For audiotapes, the school should provide written transcripts. Turning up the volume of audiotapes does not make it clearer; in fact, it often distorts the signal.

- The student's academic program should provide for two 30-minute individual sessions per week (for the regular school year and six weeks during the summer) of speech therapy and auditory training. If a speech and language pathologist, experienced in serving hearing-impaired children, is not on the school staff, the student should be seen by a certified and licensed audiologist with expertise in the educational setting.

  Moreover, if the student's evaluation determines that more specialized or intense sessions than what the in-school professional can provide are required, then the student should be referred to a clinic or private practitioner.

- There should be consistent preferential seating for the student. Depending on the room's acoustics, this may be in the front row nearest to the sound source and with the student's back to the window in order to reduce glare and improve speech reading. The audiological consultant should determine the appropriate seating position for the student.

- There should be a small number of students in the student's classes in order to minimize background noise and help the student effectively track classroom discussions. In particular, during discussions, all speakers should visually indicate that they are speaking prior to vocalizing. This would ensure that the student is facing the particular person when she or he begins to speak.

- Other necessary support services include interpreting and note-taking. CART services may also be utilized.

- There should be a consistent way of reinforcing the student's mastery of the curriculum as taught in mainstream classes. Specifically, the student should have two 30-minute sessions per week with a certified teacher of the hearing-impaired. That teacher can also act as the liaison with the mainstream classroom teacher and speech/language pathologist.

- The student's teachers should send home weekly summaries of lesson plans and include a vocabulary notebook.

- All homework assignments should be written on the blackboard or mimeograph sheet.

- The student should be included in all academic testing procedures in order to monitor progress relative to hearing peers. The student should be allowed extra time to complete exams, if necessary.

II. Regarding the Student's Social/Emotional Functioning

- Participation in a small (fewer than five peers), structured, activity-based social skills group is recommended. This would help the student learn and practice appropriate methods of socialization, particularly with regard to "picking up" those subtle social cues that are often lost in larger, mainstream settings. The group should be led by the school counselor or another appropriately trained person. If available, other hard-of-hearing peers should participate in that group.

  In this context, social skills *coaching* would be important to help the student negotiate social demands, resolve conflicts, form alliances, etc.

- A counselor—ideally the same person as in the social skills groups—should be meet with the student on a weekly basis to review whatever social issues have come up and to discuss, re-hearse, and role-play appropriate strategies. Other issues should be discussed as needed.

- A peer "mentor" may help the student learn ways of fitting in to the social milieu. This person should be a peer who is reasonably popular, "socially connected," and who would be willing and able to facilitate the student forming alliances. Naturally, the student must approve of this plan. The school counselor should monitor its implementation.

  Alternatively, it may be preferable to promote the formation of "natural" alliances. The school counselor should assess this.

- A disabilities awareness/sensitivity module for students with normal hearing may be helpful. It may help the student be more accepted by the peer network. There is probably nothing more important than to communicate well and be accepted by one's peers. Unless a child feels connected and accepted by peers, it matters relatively little how well he or she can be understood in a structured milieu.

Notes

1. Stone, D., Patton, B., & Heen, S. (1999). *Difficult conversations*. New York, NY: Viking.

CHAPTER 4

An Interrupted Story

Individually, they were nice people; but together, they turned into monsters. Tom pounded his fist on the table, throwing the coffee and accompaniments flying across the floor, and yelled at his wife, "For once in your life, shut up and listen!"

Without blinking an eye (obviously she was used to Tom's outbursts), Nancy screamed back, "You bastard! Where've you been all these years!"

"You have no right to accuse me of—"

"You talk about rights, you lousy—"

"Don't interrupt me," Tom screamed.

"Time out!" I ordered. Nancy was already waving her fist in the air.

Usually initial meetings are easy and low-key, occupied with obtaining demographic information, historical exploration and introductory descriptions of the present problem. Couples are usually on their best behavior, saving their unbridled accusations of betrayal and venomous rage for a month or so into treatment, after sufficient safety and trust have been established. Not so with Nancy and Tom. We had barely completed our initial half-hour.

However, I enjoy outbursts like these. Sometimes I imagine a full orchestra of competing instruments, each belching their tune louder than their neighbors, afraid that otherwise they would never be heard. I also think of Salvador Minuchin, my family therapist idol of sorts, who perfected the art of intervening in volatile situations forcibly yet respectfully. I learned from him that you can make interventions quite early—even ones that appear to take one side over the other—provided that you, in his words "first stroke and then kick."

The stroke: In the calmest and most authoritative voice I could muster, I looked at Tom and said, "You know, Nancy is asking a valid and important question and she deserves to know where you've been hiding, if, in fact, you have."

The kick: "But she didn't ask in a respectful way that makes it easy for you to answer." Then to Nancy, "And you, like Tom, need to learn to talk with your mouth, not your fist." Again turning toward Tom, I ended with "nevertheless, her *dis*respectfully delivered question merits a *respectful* response from you."

Tom's face was still flushed and I was unsure whether he was willing or able to back off. But he retreated surprisingly easily and abruptly shifted to a factual, almost robotic reporting of the chronology of events. He recounted that, just over 15 years ago, Alice, their then three-year-old daughter was proudly running all over the house in hot pursuit of their golden retriever who, by that time, had reconciled himself to being pursued. Alice suddenly became dizzy and lay on the couch. That night, she developed an acute fever for which the pediatrician prescribed bed rest and observation. When her fever reached over 104 degrees for the third consecutive day, she was hospitalized.

As Tom began to describe the hospital scenes, "when the doctors gave her a spinal tap and had her connected to all these machines" or "when she went in and out of consciousness," factual, robotic discourse gave way to hesitation and sorrow. He relived these traumatic memories as if they had happened yesterday, now reexperiencing their full terror in vivid colors. He looked downward, unable to complete the story.

"I can't imagine what that was like for you," I offered.

"There are no words for it," he acknowledged. "Sometime during the second night of Alice's hospitalization, I couldn't take it any longer so I split. I wandered around the streets for hours. My entire world caved in." Only moments ago, he had assaulted my coffee table and verbally abused his wife, now his manner shifted to deep despair. For the remainder of our initial 1 ½ hour meeting, Tom told the story of their daughter's meningitis, the trauma that had destroyed a significant amount of Alice's hearing and, by his account, had destroyed his marriage.

"I've never forgiven myself for those three days before she was finally hospitalized," he admitted. "Her fever kept climbing, she lost color in her face; she could hardly move her head. She was getting sicker and sicker. If only we had caught the meningitis sooner, perhaps we could have—"

"You mean if *I* caught it sooner, don't you?" Nancy interjected softly.

Tom's back arched but he then slumped in his chair. "That's part of it," he confessed.

In a meek, apologetic tone, Nancy looked at me and said, "He's always blamed me for Alice's hearing loss."

Tom and Nancy had argued briefly about insisting on a doctor's visit. At the first sign of Alice's dizziness, Tom was already mapping out the quickest route to the emergency room and practically had his coat on. Nancy, however, who was by this time used to Tom's "overreacting," convinced him to call the doctor and let her decide on the course of treatment. Tom conceded but with private misgivings. These only increased when the doctor didn't make an immediate appointment, instead adopting a wait-and-see attitude.

Tom's typical response to Nancy would have been to dig in his heels and insist on his determined course of action. In three years his stubbornness had become a frequent thorn in their marriage. Used to having his way as an only child, he had struggled with Nancy to pick his battles. He learned to concede "graciously" to Nancy's wishes about the house decor, dinner menus, etc. These struggles were all relatively unimportant, compared to the power struggles they would have in response to Alice, their first of two children. Even then, he learned to "bite his tongue" and acknowledge Nancy's authority as a coparent. But it had not come easy.

"I should have put her in the damn hospital!" Tom lamented, now slamming his fist on his knee. "But she convinced me to keep Alice at home. She told me 'Stop being an hysterical, know-it-all father; she'll be fine!' Well, she wasn't fine. She almost died. She almost died!" He screamed the last statement at Nancy, amidst tears. If looks could kill, Nancy, too, would have almost died.

"If you don't know who or what to blame, it's natural to blame yourself and/or each other," I said. It was perhaps feeble attempt to diffuse his rage. Tom did not respond. Psychologically, he had left the room, to his own private agony. I wondered what Nancy's agony was like. Turning toward her, I asked "How did your daughter's illness affect you?"

For several moments, she sat immobilized and speechless while her facial muscles contorted. Then, almost as if to supplement her nonverbal answer to my question, she kept saying, "It was horrible, it was horrible." Tom clutched the arms of his chair and Nancy followed suit.

I, too, clutched the arm of my chair. Five years prior to this meeting, my daughter almost died during childbirth. Like Tom, I still replay the doctors saying "push her out or it'll be too late" and other scenes that almost transformed the celebrated birthing process into a nightmare.

"What happens between you two when you talk about this?" I finally asked.

"We haven't," Nancy said.

"You mean you've never heard his story of what Alice's illness was like for him, and he's never heard yours?" I asked in disbelief.

Both Nancy and Tom shook their heads in shame. I didn't mean to be rudely confrontational. Indeed this kind of rigidified estrangement should not have come as a surprise. An acute, life-threatening illness of a child typically brings on a flood of intense, conflicting

and vacillating reactions for parents: grief, blame, fear, hope, closeness. If the illness results in a permanent disability, the parents' emotional instability may solidify into chronic despair and rage that first
paralyzes and then erodes and finally kills their marriage. Common
as this tragedy is, it does not have to be. I am saddened and a bit
taken aback each time I hear this familiar story.

"You're not alone in your private grief," I assured them. "It causes
many couples to feel abandoned and betrayed, precisely because the
grief is hard to talk about. By definition, it's an isolating experience."
I thought of Elie Wiesel who waited 10 years after Auschwitz before
writing his memoirs. It perhaps was not a logical free association:
equating the unfathomable Holocaust genocide to Alice's illness belittling her trauma. But a trauma story, no matter what the degree
or context, must eventually relinquish its isolating grip and be told
so that healing can begin. There is tremendous transformative power
in dialogue.

I shared with Tom and Nancy an important principle of healing:
*"The pain of loss has a size and shape, a beginning and an end. It takes
over only when not allowed its voice."*[1] The more words we have for
an experience, the more shape it has, the more it has a beginning
and end. The less words, the less space, the more it takes over."

They nodded their heads and, for an instant, looked directly at
each other. I then added, "I'm glad both of you took the brave step
of coming in."

Nancy let out a relieved smile and muttered "Thank you, Dr.
Harvey." Tom echoed her sentiment and looked toward his wife. I
responded with "you're welcome" and that they should call me
Mike. Although some people feel more comfortable addressing me
formally, it isn't my preference. After what Nancy and Tom had
shared with me, "Mike" felt more appropriate.

On the way out, Tom offered to pay for the carpet cleaning since
he had made the mess. I graciously accepted his offer. (I had
planned to give him the bill). We scheduled a meeting for the
following week.

While driving home, I replayed our initial meeting. I felt quite satisfied and even exhilarated to have so promptly interrupted their sequence of disruptive and potentially violent behaviors as well as to have excavated their underlying feelings. There is a thin line dividing rage and despair; we had explored both. That night I had a dream that Salvador Minuchin offered me lavish praise for my, in his words, "exemplary marital session." Just as we finished shaking hands goodbye and making plans to meet again soon, my alarm clock went off. A second earlier would have spoiled everything!

My psychological high lasted several days. But it was tempered by envisioning the long, difficult course of marital therapy that would surely follow. Change comes neither easily nor instantly. Couples, in particular, typically wait much too long to begin treatment. Most of us seal commitments with the unconscious hope that we will no longer have to endure remnants of childhood pain and loss. But inevitably, it's only a matter of time before we feel let down. Then one spouse may suggest getting professional help, but often the other dismisses the idea. Indeed things often improve. But if the various letdowns—disappointments, losses, betrayals, and/or trauma—are not resolved, then the marital foundation weakens, and it cannot support and resolve future misunderstandings, conflicts, and stresses that inevitably arise. Eventually, everything caves in. Unfortunately, that is when marriage counseling often begins.

Nancy and Tom were no exception to this common scenario. Alice contracting meningitis was not the first crisis in their relationship. The marriage had been beset by a host of disappointments and power struggles that began seemingly moments after they sobered up from the drunken ecstasy of falling in love. Universal in form, unique in content.

During our subsequent meetings, I learned that Nancy, as the youngest of five children, had always felt ignored and neglected by her parents. Her father was an alcoholic and kept getting laid off; her mother was chronically overwhelmed and depressed. Nancy recalled resigning herself to always getting "hand-me-downs," a status that she perceived as symbolic of her parents' indifference toward her. However, she vowed to spare her own children this fate. Tom, however, "was frugal like his father" (he was a financial planner). Tom didn't approve of buying new clothing for young children: "they don't even know the difference!" Enter Alice, 7 lbs., 4 oz. A perfect setup for heated, "life-or-death" power struggles over what she wore.

"All he would do is talk about money," Nancy complained. "He didn't get it!"

"What would have been the most empathic statement he could have made?" I asked.

"Something like 'Honey, I know it's important for you *not* to do what your parents did. So let's buy Alice some new clothes. The hell with money!'"

"And what kind of support would you have wanted from Tom when Alice was in the hospital?" On one level, this question was an abrupt change of subject from clothes to meningitis. But at another level, both of these interpersonal situations involved a labyrinth of conscious and unconscious dynamics around her thwarted hopes for Tom's empathic attunement. My question took her aback, as if she had never dared to think about it, never mind put her hopes into words in front of her husband and me. She simply said, "I don't know."

"Please speculate."

With a tentative, distant voice that hardly sounded like her own, she muttered, "For him to hold me and tell me that everything would be okay." Her eyes made fleeting contact with her husband, then darted away in fear.

"Would you say more?" I asked.

"My baby almost died for God's sake!" she cried out. But rather than escalate her fury as she had done before, Nancy now burst into tears. Then she hugged herself tightly with both arms, almost in a fetal position, and began to rock in her overstuffed chair. That was what she had needed from Tom: to be held and rocked; to be comforted and soothed; to be told that everything would be okay. In essence, she needed her husband to make up for her mother whom she had perceived as emotionally absent.

Tom, however, instead of being a surrogate mother/comforter, took the first of what would be many "walks around Boston." His methods of disengagement were to work longer hours, purportedly to "bring in more money"; to hang out with his buddies; and, as a hobby for "stress reduction," he devoted his remaining hours to becoming a wine connoisseur. He built a wine cellar, spent hours cataloging his increasing collection of varietals, joined Internet wine forums, and went to wine tastings across the country. He was well on his way to becoming a full-blown alcoholic.

Nancy felt increasingly abandoned and depressed, much like she had felt as a child. At first, she withdrew from everyone—her siblings, friends, and even Alice. But then a surprising thing happened: her mother came through for her! Nancy recalled that "for the first time I could remember, my mom was understanding and supportive. She would tell me what a good mother I was and that she was proud of me!"

On their walks and outings over coffee, Nancy's mother would vent her anger toward Tom for his emotional withdrawal. It was no secret that she had never considered him a proper son-in-law, as "he's always in his own world." At first Nancy defended Tom with "he's under a lot of stress." Like many of us, she dreaded the possibility of marrying someone like her parents, in this case, like her mother. (It was ironic that her mother's complaint about Tom's emotional unavailability echoed Nancy's complaint about her). But as Nancy felt increasingly lonely and resentful toward Tom, she joined her mother in "Tom-bashing."

In this manner, Alice's meningitis served to repair a longstanding rift between Nancy and her mother, but exacerbated the rift between Nancy and Tom.

At first, Tom was oblivious to this shifting of alliances. He was overcome by his own grief and had all he could do to get up every day, work and "support the family." I asked him when he first became aware that Nancy had emotionally left him.

In a tentative and distant voice that hardly sounded like his own, he muttered, "When I came home from work, it was like she didn't notice."

"Would you say more?" I asked.

"It was like a movie I once saw: when a guy got killed but stayed on earth as a sort-of ghost. He kept on yelling and waving to his family, but they couldn't hear or see him."

"It felt impossible for you to be heard or seen by Nancy, no matter what you did?"

"Exactly!" Tom looked out the window, struggling to hold back tears. Like Nancy, he was reexperiencing the anguish and terror that he had buried under layers of defenses.

"What did you need from her when you came home?" I gently persisted.

A simple question in the abstract, but one that apparently had never been asked. Consequently, it crumbled his defenses. His body contorted in a holding-on-for-dear-life position; his mouth quivered in tormented pain, and tears ran down his face He cried out, "I only wanted her to hug me, like she used to."

I followed a hunch, "And to be told that everything is okay, to be comforted and soothed?"

"Yes, yes!" Tom cried. An amazing, but to many therapists, no longer surprising phenomenon: Nancy's and Tom's needs and wants were mirror images of each other. Both needed the other to be a soothing, all-knowing, all-comforting parent; instead, they experienced the other as inflicting cruel abandonment.

However, as we walked through the chronology, I could see their toxic patterns beginning to shift. Now, as Tom's emotional pain finally became visible to Nancy, she leaned forward toward him. Tom, in turn, made eye contact with her. I imagined the beginnings of a resurrected love that had seemed dead for many years.

We were on a roll. It would now be important to explore the

origins of Tom's feeling abandoned by a loved one as a first step in helping him separate past from present emotional reactions. I asked him whether he had felt feelings of abandonment in his childhood. He readily volunteered a childhood memory.

> "When I was a seven-year-old kid, I was roller skating around the neighborhood after supper and fell down. My knee was bleeding all over the road. I lay there crying my eyes out but no one came. I guess my mom came only a few minutes later; but back then it seemed like an eternity."

"And then what happened?"

"She took me home and bandaged me up."

The "eternity" of waiting for his mother didn't seem quite severe enough to explain Tom's report of having felt emotionally abandoned. I wondered about the role that his father played. "Was your dad home?" I asked.

"Yeah."

"And what did he do?"

Tom hesitated and then averted eye contact with me: "He told me not to cry, to be a man."

"And how did that feel?"

"I felt ashamed, but I was scared of bleeding to death! He wasn't there for me."

"In addition to you feeling abandoned, he essentially taught you to deal with crises by taking walks, working, drinking wine, hiding—anything except showing your pain?"

A pause. "Yeah, I guess so." Tom's eyes met mine. He made the connection. As our time was up, we scheduled our next meeting.

They began the hour by recounting how Alice's hearing loss had been diagnosed at the age of four, several months after she had contracted meningitis. Although all the doctors gave firm assurances that she had made a complete recovery and that there would be no residual complications, Nancy and Tom noticed that she didn't respond as quickly to directions and that she more frequently lost her balance when chasing the dog. They became concerned.

One morning, after Nancy noticed once again that Alice was having difficulty understanding her speech, she called the pediatrician to authorize a hearing test. The doctor was busy and would call back. However, this time, Nancy, politely but firmly, told the receptionist to interrupt her and get immediate authorization. Nancy, too, had berated herself for having much earlier abided by the doctor's wait-and-see attitude. She would wait no more. She got an appointment with an audiologist for that afternoon.

Nancy called Tom at work with the hope that he would accompany her. However, he could not make the appointment because of "a prior business commitment." Nancy went with her mother instead. After a thorough evaluation and review of the history, the audiologist rendered a diagnosis of "a moderate, downward sloping, bilateral, sensori-neural hearing loss, presumably secondary to meningitis." Alice's audiogram and speech reception thresholds revealed a moderate hearing loss in the lower frequencies, sloping to a severe-to-profound loss in the higher frequencies in both ears, which meant she found it easier to understand men's voices than women's and children's voices. Nancy recalled thinking what a cruel irony it was that, in light of Tom's previous absenteeism, Alice would have less difficulty understanding him than she would Nancy.

The audiologist, obviously knowledgeable about psychological and family dynamics, did not simply send Nancy and her mother on their way. Not only did she give them relevant literature and information about support groups, but she emphasized to Nancy that "It would be very important for you *and your husband* to completely understand everything." Thus, the audiologist scheduled a follow-up appointment with both of them. Nancy recalled being impressed that she "seemed to have an intuition that things weren't okay with my marriage."

Nancy told me that, much to her delight, Tom made it to the next meeting, asked many questions, and took copious notes. The audiologist again explained the ramifications of hearing loss and also told them that meningitis sometimes causes learning disabilities.

She recommended later psychological or neuropsychological testing for Alice. In the middle of giving her chronology, Nancy glanced at Tom and me, and shared a spontaneous insight: "It's weird to say this, but that time was one of the happiest of our marriage! I got my husband back!" But in reaction to Nancy's insight, Tom looked down, perhaps in boredom or in shame, I could not tell which. When I asked him what he was thinking, he replied "nothing."

Again their relationship showed vacillating closeness and distance. Where earlier I sensed a renewed connection between them—what I perhaps prematurely considered resurrected love—now I sensed renewed disengagement, anger, betrayal, and despair. It felt like an odd juxtaposition to witness their increasingly embittered disengagement as Nancy recounted their past renewed intimacy.

Nancy sighed deeply and continued her chronology. "Tom and I united over our daughter's special needs. We learned about hearing aids, speech therapy and Public Law 94-142 (Individuals with Disabilities Education Act). We wanted to make sure that Alice would receive enough support services at our local school. We ended up getting her an FM system, speech therapy, and occupational therapy to help her with balance problems. And we even got the school to install rugs and acoustic tiles."

At first, Nancy found solace in Tom's ardent efforts to learn about hearing loss and its remediation. For Tom, unlike the amorphousness of meningitis, the concreteness of the audiogram with its hearing thresholds, speech discrimination scores, etc., gave him a *raison d'etre,* a passion beyond what he could get by dallying in wine tasting. He felt that finding a cure for Alice's hearing impairment would be the means of "cutting out" and expelling his rage and guilt for having waited those three precious days before hospitalizing Alice.

He brought home reams of articles from the library about advanced hearing aid technology or future prospects for artificial implants. (This was before cochlear implants became popular.) He read through countless alternative medicine journals in search of an herb, an elixir, a remedy—anything that might somehow restore Alice's hearing. Nancy and Tom read these articles together. And spurred on by their new found intimacy around Alice, they conceived a second child.

But ultimately, Tom's psychological scalpel for removing his psychic pain was woefully inadequate. If only it were that simple. Nancy confirmed that "After a while, something happened. He went back to his old self, became distant, drank too much, and became hostile again. When he wasn't hiding behind alcohol, he would explode at me." She clenched her fist, then let it drop in her lap. Her posture portrayed a mixture of barely contained protest and resignation.

Tom began to squirm in his seat, much like I remembered him doing on our very first visit before he assaulted my coffee table. I asked him to reflect on what he did with his anger toward himself for purportedly failing to prevent Alice's hearing loss; and what he did with his anger at Nancy for the same. Maybe reflection and processing would help avoid another explosion.

Much to my relief, his body became still. Then after a moment of reflection, he responded with "Maybe I was so pissed off at her that I really did go back into hiding by drinking too much."

Tom was half-right; in my view, he *never stopped hiding.* The only difference was that after he initially cut down on his drinking, he used a different hiding place: libraries instead of wine tastings. And when he was not hiding, he was explosive toward Nancy.

Another amazing but not surprising phenomena: Whenever we are cut off from some part of ourselves, we suffer an inner conflict that will inevitably take the form of outer conflict with those we love.[2] What we cannot tolerate in ourselves, we act out with our partners. It was not a coincidence that Nancy was "pissed off" at Tom for his "negligent, spineless, selfish hiding." Her criticisms of Tom were identical to those criticisms that he (largely unconsciously) levied against himself. Tom unconsciously engineered it so that the disowned parts of himself—"the spineless wimp"—would come from Nancy as an accusation against him. He would therefore be spared of consciously experiencing significant internal self-loathing; it would come out of Nancy's mouth, not his. As he told me many years later in retrospect, he eventually figured out that he, in fact, felt ashamed of "wimping out and hiding"—albeit below his conscious awareness—even while doing his research on hearing loss.

It was also no coincidence that Tom's explosive criticisms of Nancy echoed his self-criticisms. Since he could not tolerate his own guilt-laden feelings of self-loathing, he not only experienced them as coming from Nancy—so-called "projection"—but he also discharged his anger and loathing onto Nancy. Via both of these complex psychological mechanisms, he could get "pissed off" at *her,* as if the "beast" was part of her—"What a bitch!"—as opposed to it being part of him. I'm okay; you're not okay.

Tom was not the only culpable party; a dance requires partners. Nancy, too, had tried in vain to cut out and expel the parts of herself that she found intolerable, most notably her childhood feelings of second-hand status and expecting only fleeting bits of love and attention. But like all of us, she discovered that by trying to simply expiate herself of her vulnerabilities, she acted them out instead. In her own words, "Now I realize that I should have insisted that Tom cancel his goddamn office appointment and go with me to the audiologist. But I acted like I deserved whatever scraps I got."

Nancy was not the originator of this imagery. Her muted rage and shame had their roots in her mother's feelings of resigned entrapment by her alcoholic husband; she, too, felt like she deserved only scraps. It was no wonder then that Nancy and her mother rebonded as coconspirators against Tom. The rage that Nancy expressed toward Tom was what her mother had been unable to express toward her own husband.

"It all seems so clear in retrospect," Nancy and Tom agreed.

"It always is. But you're quickly becoming more adept at catching yourself becoming entrapped by the labyrinth," I emphasized. Indeed, they were making good progress.

As we continued to meet on a weekly basis, Tom and Nancy gradually became more able to look at these complex layers of personal and couple dynamics without becoming overwhelmed by them and without acting them out on each other. They took initial steps toward forgiving themselves, which served as a foundation for them to truly forgive each other. Things were going well.

Often they would lament over "lost time." This is a normal and healthy kind of grieving process where one reconciles the "what if" questions. What if Nancy and Tom had not taken so many "walks" away from each other? What would have happened if, instead, they had used the crises of Alice's meningitis as an opportunity—a critical juncture—to openly mourn together? What if they had sought help much earlier? What if they hadn't expected their marriage to resolve their individual issues? What if...?

"If only we knew then what we know now," Nancy lamented. Tom nodded his head.

"The show's not over," I responded. "Some people never get to where you've worked so hard to be. You should be very proud of yourselves. Yes, grieve the loss but look forward to a deeper, more meaningful, happier future. And you'll also be able to teach your kids what your parents weren't able to teach you." Alice was now 17 years old and their son, Alex, was entering adolescence.

Tom and Nancy smiled. She accepted her husband's outstretched hand. Their eyes connected solidly, as if to acknowledge their deepening love for each other, particularly in light of the hard work they had done. Undoubtedly this would be the first of many steps they would take toward each other. We made another appointment for a month.

***

On a warm, sunny morning after our meeting, I began my usual ritual of making coffee and reading the paper. Soon I would water my garden. But then my ritual was interrupted. The headlines had to be wrong. There must be several Nancy Downing's in the Boston area. The Nancy I knew had to have been home with her kids, with her husband, at work, out shopping, walking the dog—anywhere except in a fatal car accident. But my phone call to their home confirmed my worst fears. After introducing myself, I asked whether I could talk to Nancy. Nancy was dead.

As I write this chapter, I am very tempted to omit this part. Why depress the reader? Why not end this story on a happy, upbeat note? Nancy and Tom holding hands, making love, walking their children down the aisle at their weddings, having grandchildren. This ending is not fair to the reader, to me, and, of course, most of all, to Nancy, Tom, and their children whose lives were brutally interrupted. God knows, they should have been rewarded with a far better ending for their hard work.

It has been several years since Nancy's death. I often find myself asking modified versions of my earlier "what if" questions: What if they somehow knew that Nancy would soon die? Would they have wasted so much time hiding from each other? Would they have be more able to relish every day, every minute of their marriage—"til death do us part"—as they (like most of us) promised at the alter?

All our maneuvers to avoid intimacy, our marital tiffs, our arguments and power struggles suddenly appear petty, grossly unnecessary. The lesson becomes so clear. But then come more questions: Do we humans, for some reason, *have to* continually 'work through' endless layers of our pettiness in order to transcend a fear of intimacy? Must we strive to complete our story that, by design, must remain *in*complete? Does our personal, marital, and spiritual growth come down to this paradox?

I would never have wished that their marriage ended so tragically. But of course I do not have the power to change such fundamental endings; only to engage in the persistent struggle to illuminate those existential possibilities that we have between the beginning and the end.

My temptations for omission aside, the ending of An Interrupted Story must remain as is. It's honest. It's ethical. And more importantly, Nancy's cruel and tragic death contains vital life-giving lessons that, through our sadness, outrage and grieving, we can at least try to understand. With personal reflection and interpersonal dialogue, we can attempt to answer those unanswerable questions of life and love.

Notes

1. Brener, A., Riemer, J., & Cutter, W. (1993). *Mourning and mitzvah: A guided journal for walking the mourner's path through grief and healing.* Vermont: Jewish Lights.
2. Welwood, J. (1996). *Love and awakening: Discovering the sacred path of intimate relationship.* New York: HarperPerrenial.

CHAPTER 5

The Soulful Biologist

George's world seemed different than mine. It contained discrete bits of data, inventories of biological phenomena, and epidemiological statistics of animal and plant species around the world, complete with their scientific names. He would point out different kinds of plants around us: a Disentra, Pinquicula, Nasturium, Nautilocalyx, to mention only a few. I would nod my head politely.

I first met George at a week-long conference held at a beautiful convention center on the grounds of a national forest and seashore. We were on a panel together to speak about the effects of hearing loss; my talk would be from a professional perspective, his from a personal perspective. Now in his early 60s, he had a gradually deteriorating hearing loss, first noticeable to others when he was 50 years old, and, at least on a conscious level, to himself a few years later. He had recently retired from a research position as a senior biologist at a prestigious university.

His lecture struck me as an odd mixture of irrelevant and inspirational. It had nothing to do with hearing loss and I wondered why he was chosen for the panel. He told the audience that although he classified himself as "mildly hard-of-hearing," he had never seen an audiologist and considered his impaired hearing "superfluous." "It didn't matter; there are more important things in life." He then gave a sermon on retirement. For over a half hour, he covered the importance of financial planning, keeping active, learning about "the world we live in" and being frugal with resources. He proudly gave a step-by-step description of how he had changed the plumbing in his toilets to use 25% less water per flush. Less ecological waste; more savings in water bills. People in the audience were taking notes.

Afterward, he invited me out for a walk. After giving the scientific names for the umpteenth bush, tree, shrub, and plant, he defined what he termed the most amazing phenomenon on earth: *photosynthesis.* "It is the process by which chlorophyll-containing organisms, such as green plants, capture energy in the form of light and convert it to chemical energy. Virtually all the energy available for life in the earth's atmosphere is made available through photosynthesis. There's nothing like it in all the world," he said. I nodded my head.

His jokes weren't bad—mostly corny sexual puns. It was odd, though, how he interspersed them in his tutorials, almost as non sequiturs. After a joke, George would laugh and his face would flush a bit. I laughed, too; sometimes because the joke was humorous, other times because it gave me welcome respite. A minute later—no more!—he would return to describing the ecological environment. He was a well-oiled human machine with an insatiable craving for information.

Apparently, his three children were also recipients of George's pedagogy. He told me how important it had been to teach them about the world, so "they wouldn't end up ignorant like most people—enslaved and trapped in their own limited bubbles." His quest had an *Exodus*-like feel to it (reminiscent to me of the Jewish Passover that ritualizes Jews' liberation from the entrapment of Egypt), but compulsive. Over a decade later, his son would tell me how George had forced the family to travel in the car for hours, days, weeks—with minimal breaks and only to use the bathrooms, get food, and sleep—in order to experience, first hand, a piece of nature or man-made structure. His modus operandi seemed in marked contrast to John Steinbeck's wisdom, in *Travels With Charlie,* that the *process* of traveling is more important than arriving at the final destination.[1] For George, the destination was everything.

The conference was coming to an end and I was looking forward to returning to the routine of my life. A week was enough, both of the conference and of George. Defensive at first, I thought that perhaps I deprived myself of new ways of experiencing the surroundings that he had to offer. Then I reminded myself that, for the first several hours, I was quite appreciative of his teachings. But there was a reason why I became a psychologist rather than a biologist.

After we finished packing our cars, George approached me and shook my hand warmly, in an almost uncharacteristically intimate manner, as if he was acknowledging a budding affection and the beginnings of a long friendship. He made solid eye contact with me and, for an instant, it looked like he held back tears. It took me aback. Now I felt a bit cheated, as if I'd been allowed to see only a fleeting glimpse of what lay underneath his armor. I had the sense that he was besieged by an onerous fear that caused him to retreat to a private citadel, the boundaries of which perhaps only he knew. We exchanged a fond goodbye.

Ten years later he telephoned me. "I'm flying into the Boston area for a meeting until next week and I would appreciate your professional advice on something. But if you can't fit me in, I'll understand. I know you're busy."

I saw him the next day. After exchanging a warm handshake, I beckoned him into my office. He had aged much more than a decade, now looking older than his 73 years. I sensed something was wrong, perhaps health-related issues or family problems. But I couldn't resist an affectionate jab before we would get down to business.

"Did you notice my plant over there? It's a *Venus vinfintoris!*" (It sounded Latin enough to me).

"You should water it more," George retorted. We both laughed.

"Well, again thank you very much for seeing me, Mike."

"It's my pleasure, George. What's new with you?"

"Well, I'm losing more hearing and find that I miss things more than I used to. I'm doing okay with it, though. And hearing aids are so expensive, over $3000 someone told me! What I do is concentrate more on what people are saying and it's okay most of the time."

"Uh huh," I responded, inviting him to continue.

"I'm on a committee and we're planning several meetings on hybrid development—a cross between maple and oak—that would result in both a decreased fire hazard due to the deciduous nature of the trees and increased wood production, which is stronger and more durable than what is presently produced. You see, now..."

A déjà vu. This time, however, our meeting was on my turf. So I interrupted him with "George, I'm glad to see you. But you didn't come here to tell me all this. What's going on?"

"Well, yeah that's true. Uh, well, I'm wondering what advice or articles you have about how hearing-impaired people, particularly older people like me, can hear better at these meetings I'm setting up. I know that you know a lot about that kind of technology."

"Actually, I don't. As a psychologist, I can talk with you about emotional issues of hearing loss, coping strategies, et cetera. But I know some very good audiologists who know a lot about what acoustic modifications you can make at meetings or conferences. I'd be happy to refer you to them," I offered.

"Yes, that would be helpful. I would appreciate that."

"At the same time, you also really owe it to yourself to get a good hearing evaluation and for an audiologist to walk you through what would help you to hear better."

"I suppose it can't hurt," he replied.

"Good. But please, George, as long as you're here, tell me how you've been. How's your health? How's your family?" I had a suspicion that he hadn't come to me for audiological advice.

As if he was waiting for me to ask, he promptly disclosed his real anguish: "Well, I've had medical problems. I've been in a lot of pain and no doctor has been able to diagnose what's going on." His face grimaced a bit and I got my first glimpse of his fear. George explained that, several years ago, he had first suffered from severe gastro-intestinal distress, so much that he could hardly sleep.

"I'm very sorry to hear how much pain you're in. What do you think's going on?" I was still unclear why he opted to come see *me* at this particular time.

"Frankly, Mike, I don't know why I'm in pain or really why I'm here. You don't prescribe medicine, I know that; and you're not about to do more tests on me. But my oldest son has been cutting out newspaper articles about biofeedback and stress reduction and has been after me to do it. Maybe you know something about that and can give me some references?"

"I'd be happy to give you some leads about stress reduction. Tell me, though, what's your son most concerned about?" I asked.

"He thinks I'm depressed, but I hardly ever see him." An uncharacteristically abbreviated and somber reply. I found myself wondering what George's relationship with his son was like. There was a sense of sadness that came through, perhaps a longing for closeness that I, too, had sensed many years ago with us.

"Please say more."

"Like he thinks this pain is all in my head." He shook his head several times, seemingly in resignation.

There is a Yiddish word, *souris,* which means sorrow or suffering. I sensed George's souris. Perhaps it was a direct result of his current physical distress; but, on reflection, it seemed longstanding. I flashed back to our goodbye at the conference, to what was left *un*-said between us, as if he wanted to say so much more, leaving me, and perhaps also him, feeling cheated. Many questions to explore.

"It sounds like you notice more the pain in your gut, not in your head," I responded. "But the body is a sort of biological/psychological ecosystem: what's going on in your head is often felt in your gut." I used his personal, biological metaphors, but was afraid they might take us away from exploring his emotional world. Maybe we could do both.

"George, do *you* think you're depressed?" I asked.

"Well, I certainly get tired a lot, but that's because I can't sleep for more than a couple of hours. It's also because I have to strain to hear people and have to do a lot of lipreading. My doctor has run a lot of tests, like..." Having ever so briefly hinted at depression, he was now running like hell in the opposite direction. In his characteristic scientific manner, he listed the complete regimen of diagnostic procedures. Inasmuch as he was brilliant and erudite about the world outside of him, he was naive and frightened about his inner world. Psychotherapy never occurred to him. Perhaps it was never suggested.

His request of me, however, was for articles on stress reduction and biofeedback, not therapy. But I was struck by what may have been his *non*verbal SOS signal emanating from an inner grimace that I imagined hammered against his skull, causing his forehead to squint tight. He seemed lonely and in mourning, as if he had been cheated out of a cherished something or someone. Simply giving him clinical information and bidding him goodbye would have honored his verbal request, but would have ignored perhaps a much more ephemeral, hidden request. Hopefully, the unspoken but intimate connection that I sensed we both felt would guide the next step. I took the leap.

"George, of course, I'd be happy to copy some materials for you. But, if you have time now, can we talk a bit about you, your life, sort of switch gears a bit and help me get to know a more personal part of you?" As luck would have it, my next hour was free.

"What do you mean?" he asked.

"I know you didn't explicitly say you're coming here for psychotherapy, but maybe we can make this a sort of introductory session. What do you think?"

"What exactly is psychotherapy?" he asked. "Old scientists like me don't know a hell of a lot about that stuff." His admission didn't surprise me. It contained elements of resignation and fear.

An abrupt shift: "*Alchemy* is an ancient art devoted chiefly to

transmuting common metals into gold," I began, slowly and rhyth-
mically, while maintaining eye contact with George. In reaction to
my non sequitur, his eyes dilated a bit and he leaned forward in his
chair. Knowing that I now had a sure audience, albeit a confused
one, I continued.

> The fundamental concept of alchemy was that all things tend to
> reach perfection. Because other metals were thought to be less "perfect"
> than gold, it was reasonable to assume that nature formed gold out of those
> metals and that, with sufficient skill and diligence, an artisan could dupli-
> cate this process in the workshop.

"But alchemy turned out to be bogus," George interrupted. He
easily engaged in this academic discourse.

"That's true," I replied. "But unlike photosynthesis, its truth lies
not in the concrete phenomenon, but in its metaphorical value."

"What do you mean?"

"I mean we have the capacity to transmute common events—
'common metals'—in our lives into something transformative,
into gold."

Again George returned only a confused stare. This is progress, I
thought, since it was the antithesis of him lecturing me. I told him
the story of Primo Levi, a chemist who was imprisoned by the Nazis.
He used the transmutability of the elements as a metaphor to explain how he withstood his torture. When he was close to despair
and considering giving in to death, he took care to wash his face
every day. It was one volitional act that he, and *he alone,* could control. Thus, this ordinary act became *extraordinary;* it turned into
gold; and it restored dignity and structure to his person.[2]

"Maybe you can transmute your physical pain into gold," I said.

"Good, then I can invest it in mutual funds," he joked, but in an
obviously sarcastic and dismissive manner. Then he became more
direct: "I want my stomach pain to go away! It prevents me from
sleeping!"

"I very much hope it goes away, too, George. It keeps you up at night; it sounds like it's excruciating. You're correctly trying to do everything in your power to get rid of it. But you're stuck with the pain, at least for now. So what's the opportunity here; where's the gold?"

In response to him shrugging his shoulders, I persevered. "You know, George, you've busted your ass over the years to teach your then young children to appreciate common artifacts of the world. Do you think that you have nothing else to teach them? Pain of one kind or another is at least as common as artifacts or trees. Maybe you could use your stomach pain as a springboard to teach your children important lessons about life, perhaps about how to deal with loss, fear, uncertainty. You know, your words 10 years ago made a big impression on me: that you don't want them to end up 'ignorant like most people—enslaved and trapped in their own limited bubbles.' Remember you telling me that? Your kids will have similar pain someday and they'll need to know from you what the hell to do with it."

My speech struck a nerve. George had always spent much time worrying about his kids, although it seemed that he never told them that. In a moment of raw honesty, he sighed, "I don't know how to talk with them. They talk to their mother, not to me."

"Like there's a distance between you?"

"Yeah," he said in a long sigh, while nodding his head.

George had taken the leap with me. Perhaps we could now explore where the distance and estrangement with his kids came from. "This pattern usually has a history to it, often from previous generations. Tell me, how did you talk with your own parents?"

"I didn't," he replied instantly. Now leaning forward in his chair—as if the door to his personal background had swung open—George told me some of his story: "I was the only child of working class parents on a farm in Nebraska. My dad was a machinist and my mother a housewife. When I was 12 years old, my father died from an ulcer. My mother and I did the best we could, struggling to make ends meet. School was my escape, as I had always done well academically. I excelled at sports and was an avid member of the debating team and science club."

"Your father died from an ulcer?" I asked.

"He didn't have to die," George recollected. "But he never went to the doctor and ended up bleeding internally. He literally bled to death."

"Why do you think he didn't go the doctor?"

"I don't rightly know. He didn't trust doctors. And he was an eternal optimist, I suppose. Always thought that everything would somehow turn out all right. He was a dreamer."

"He messed that up, didn't he?"

"Sure did," George sighed.

"Permit me to ask you this: what lesson did that teach you?"

"Lesson?"

"Lesson about how to live your own life, what to teach your children."

"Take care of things, learn everything you can about the world, be prepared for the future, use energy wisely. I have a Toyota that has over 200,000 miles on it! I change the oil myself every 3000 miles, change the spark plugs, and am always sure to change the air cleaner and carburetor settings. All my tools stay organized in boxes, away from the humidity and heat so they don't warp. I use rechargeable batteries as much as possible, which saves energy. And I make sure to store my hearing aids in low-humidity containers that I made myself."

Again, we got a bit too close to his pain, I thought. However, on an externalized, symbolic level, he was very much answering my question: he lost his dad because he hadn't properly taken care of himself; now George diligently learned about and took care of his Toyota, hearing aids, and other possessions to keep them alive so that they, too, wouldn't betray him. He painstakingly took care of objects in his external world in order to escape the souris within his soul. It invited further exploration.

"Your dad left you at a critical time, right before your adolescence."

"Yep."

"Could you expand that 'Yep' a little?"

George gave a wry smile and expanded it a token amount: "It was hard but we persevered."

"Your mother and you?"

"Uh huh."

"Yep," I smiled.

He smiled back somewhat anxiously. I now became quiet, opting not to chase him, but to allow him to take the next step in our dialogue. In contrast to his previous pontifications about photosynthesis, waste disposal systems, etc., now George's verbal output was sparse. I had an image of his door slamming shut. His countenance, however, gave away his secret; it was a secret that perhaps even he was not privy to. Whereas he typically did not display much emotion, except when talking about photosynthesis, etc., now he looked sullen and somber.

"It was hard," he finally said. It was a reiteration of what he had just said, but this time filled with deep sadness.

Boys need their fathers to become men. In the words of psychiatrist Frank Pittman, "We [men] long for our father. We wear his clothes, and actually try to fill his shoes. Anything of his is charmed and can endow us with his masculinity. We spend so much more time with our mother we begin to fear she will stifle the masculinity we know we must develop in ourselves... Every boy must have a man who is rooting [for him]."[3]

The unexpected death of George's father undoubtedly left him feeling cheated, flooded with grief and terrified. But like many men of his and my generation, he learned that the "mature" response to loss is to grit your teeth and bear it. John Wayne. But pain doesn't go away; it only gets transformed. It became clear that George's primal fear was the loss or stifling of his own vitality, his own manhood; and that this fear manifested itself as almost compulsive rituals of learning about and taking care of material possessions so that he wouldn't lose them, too.

His mother tried the best she could to be both a mom and dad. But she couldn't do it alone. George described her as "very driven and very strict," traits that increased in severity after his father's death. I imagined that these traits were her home-made tactics for "rooting for his masculinity," implemented at the expense of showing George her soft, feminine side, or *anima*. I tried to imagine what it must have been like for his mom to lose the one person whom George needed to become a man.

"In what way was she strict?" I asked.

"She would examine the minute details of everything I did—homework, cleaning up, fixing things around the house, sports—and would criticize me for what I did wrong and lecture me how I could do better next time. Nothing could satisfy her."

"Why do you think she became like that?" I asked.

"I don't know."

"Speculate."

"Well, I suppose she was trying to prepare me for the world, for how to take care of myself."

"Take care of yourself how?"

"Study hard, learn as much as you can, work hard, and save money."

"And whatever you do, don't be optimistic," I remarked.

"Uh huh," George said. "For the last years of her life (she died a few months before you and I met at that conference) she was losing her hearing and withdrew from everybody. She had advanced arthritis as well and had trouble moving."

"She let her hearing loss and physical pain create a distance between her and you."

"Yeah, she complained about muffled sounds and not being able to understand. She was a world all her own."

"Which didn't include you; which didn't allow for her to teach you even more lessons about life, namely how to deal with pain and loss. Both of you had progressive hearing losses."

"You're right about that!" George said clearly, now with a bit more fervor.

"You don't want to replicate that pattern with your kids, do you?"

A pause. "No, I don't." This time, George smiled. He could see where I was going, and then he surprised me. After another hesitation, he looked at me and said, "I've told my oldest son about you as he's the one who wanted me to see somebody. Can we come in for a meeting together?"

This time it was me who hesitated. To save myself from disappointment, I have learned not to necessarily count on my therapeutic hopes really being actualized. I thought to myself that it's a dream come true: first photosynthesis, gastrointestinal distress, Toyota engine maintenance, loss of father and mother and now him working on his relationship with his son! I am continually amazed when things actually go as planned.

"It would be my absolute pleasure." We made an appointment for a few days.

Larry didn't look at all like his father. A handsome, middle-aged man, he was short in stature with eyes that burst with passion. His face easily revealed a rich emotional life and exuberance. He claimed to have inherited his mother's sensitivity to people and his father's appreciation of knowledge. His career was as a counselor for disabled people in the Boston area.

As George had requested the meeting, I looked to him to begin.

"Well, uh, Larry says he's worried about me, but he doesn't need to be."

"I am worried about you, dad," he said directly to George. "I'm worried that you do nothing and that you're wasting away. I'm worried that you're getting poor medical care and taking too many pills."

"Is your worst fear that he'll end up like your grandfather?" I interjected.

It was the albatross that they hadn't acknowledged. After a pause, Larry replied, "That's *exactly* what I'm worried about." Then Larry looked at George and cried, "I'm afraid you'll drop dead!"

A poignant moment that I let linger. Then I broke the silence: "You know, I have a strong hunch that there's a lot of important things both of you haven't said to each other and that it'll take some time. I don't want to begin something and then prematurely say good-bye. Can we agree on perhaps a few more meetings before we continue this conversation?" Before I attempted to unearth the toxins that lay buried in their relationship, it would be important to ensure that we would have a minimum number of sessions to work it through. George and Larry agreed to four meetings. We could now proceed.

To Larry, I said "I do think we should talk about how your dad is or is not taking care of himself, but permit me, if you will, to point to another related issue, albeit a difficult one to talk about." I turned my head to George: "You know, it's a reality that sooner or later all of us, including you, will die. You were telling me earlier that there are some things you want to tell your son before that happens. What do you most want to say to him?"

George thought for a long moment. Again, his eyes showed the impassioned, almost tormented, part of him that I had glimpses of before. But now his desperate yearning for an intimate bond with Larry, something that he had never had with either of his parents, became dominant.

"That I love him, that I think about him a lot, that I worry and hope he'll be okay."

"Would you say that to him?"

He looked at Larry, then at me: "That he—"

"Look at him. 'That you—'"

"That you take care of things, invest and save your money, and don't—"

"Dad, you've told me all that before," Larry interrupted with mild annoyance.

"It's easier for your dad to give advice, to keep his feelings to himself or to reveal them during goodbyes," I suggested.

Larry emphatically nodded his head.

I then took a different tack. I asked George to portray their relationship by positioning himself and Larry in my office at a certain distance from each other, with specific body postures, and so on. This is a well-known technique called *sculpting*. It is a compact, powerful way of summarizing a lot of verbal material in nonverbal portraits.

With some coaxing and several demonstrations, George was able to set up his sculpture. After positioning Larry, he moved a standing light fixture next to him to represent his wife. He placed himself at the opposite end of the room and he looked longingly toward Larry, with one hand outstretched toward him and his other hand placed on his forehead in confusion. When asked what his associated thoughts were, he lamented, "I don't know what to say to him."

"Do you know what they're talking about?" I asked.

"I have no idea! I can't understand a word they're saying!"

"You're able to hear that they're talking about something but it's all mumbles?"

"Yeah!"

Now Larry yelled "Why didn't you say something, Dad? Why didn't you say 'I can't understand what you two are talking about. Would you tell me? I wanna join in.' Why do you just stand there?"

George responded in resignation, "I don't know. I'm sorry, I'm very sorry."

There was a long pause. My mind jumped to the many elderly persons who have lost a significant amount of hearing and have withdrawn from their world and family. But it is always more complex than that. Now I asked Larry to sculpt how he had often felt with his father. He, too, placed both himself and George on opposites sides of the room. Larry then stooped on the floor and outstretched his arms toward his father while looking slightly away from him. He stood George up on a chair and depicted him as pointing toward some scenery in the distance. He did not depict his mother at all. Larry's associated thoughts were, "I want to be much closer to Dad but he hardly notices me." His voice cracked and tears rolled down his cheeks. George looked heartbroken, confused, and desperately lost.

"Larry, can I ask you to put into words what has been the most difficult thing to talk about between you and your dad, what has kept you emotionally on opposite sides of the room for so long?"

He hesitated, seemingly because I was asking him to break a rule about not criticizing George to his face. But after George assured him that it was okay—in his words, "I'm a big boy now"—Larry took the risk and provided a compact yet potent summary statement of his childhood relationship with him: "It always had to be his way. I could do nothing right."

Larry shared his recollections about how the family was frequently subjected to George's rage and panic that something bad would happen if they didn't behave in a precisely prescribed way. His most vivid childhood memory was when he and his dad were walking their dog on the beach: "Without warning, dad yelled, 'Pull the dog in!' with explosive rage, and screamed that if the dog had scratched someone, we could be sued and lose everything." As a child, Larry did not have the cognitive–emotional tools to understand that George was anxious and fearful. He naturally interpreted his action as once again indicating that he could do nothing right.

Because of how George expressed his love and concern for his children, it seemed that they viewed him as a tyrant. He alone would design the itinerary for excursions in order to maximize the educational exposure for the kids; he would strictly limit how long the kids spent in direct sunlight for fear of them getting skin cancer; and he would closely ensure that the kids always had impeccably balanced meals—breakfast, lunch, and dinner.

George helplessly looked down toward the floor. I turned to Larry. "It sounds like your dad was desperately trying to prevent Armageddon." It was time to begin reframing George as a fearful and desperate man instead of a tyrant.

Larry nodded his head. Having gone to psychotherapy himself several years prior, he slowly came to realize that his dad had always been afraid and insecure. "I've always kind of known that," he said. "And losing his hearing seemed to make him even more anxious."

"Did he lecture more as he lost more hearing?" I asked.

"Yeah, he sure did," Larry replied without missing a beat.

Again, a familiar scenario. I speculated that George lectured more in order to spare himself the anxiety and perhaps humiliation of not understanding what was being said. But, at the same time, since he could not control his progressive hearing loss, it led to increasing anxiety; and in turn, he lectured more. A vicious cycle.

Predictably, George was taking Larry's barrage of disclosures very hard. I took a stab at reading his mind, as it was an easy guess: "George, if I were you, I'd probably feel like a failure as a father, guilty, ashamed, and so on. Am I right?"

He nodded his head, this time understandably choosing not to speak. I encouraged him to put his feelings into words.

"Mike, for the life of me, I honestly don't know what to say. I don't know the words; I wish I did. I never wanted to do anything to hurt him!" Now George's voice cracked, much like his son's had only a few minutes ago.

"George. Move time backward 60 years. Seems like a hell of a long time for me, but I bet, in some ways, it seems like a blink of an eye to you. What would you have liked your dad to have said to you if you hadn't been cheated of so much time with him?"

A simple but complicated question. He looked stunned and a bit shaken up. But then he became quite still and I sensed his answer churning within him.

"George," I said, now making direct eye contact with him, "Would you tell your son the answer to my question: what you wanted and needed from your dad."

George nodded his head and made eye contact with his son

whom he had cherished at a distance for so many years. He said softly and slowly, "I wanted my dad to be my friend." He paused, looked away but then looked back into Larry's eyes. "And I want that for us. I want you to be my friend."

Between tears, Larry held out his hands and clasped his dad's hands, holding them tightly and lovingly. "I want that, too, Dad." Many moments passed.

Breaking the silence, George read my mind: "It's made of the same stuff, isn't it?"

"What do you mean?" I asked.

"What I needed from my dad is what Larry needed from me!"

"He still needs those things from you."

"I know," George responded. Larry nodded.

Until now, George had encoded his thwarted relationship with his father as separate from his thwarted relationship with his son. Separated by a time span of over 60 years, one obviously had nothing to do with the other. But he was beginning to see them as interconnected, as "made of the same stuff." Consequently, he realized new possibilities for himself, for his son and for their relationship. They sat silently for another moment, letting it all sink in.

I couldn't help but be fascinated how the almost magical transformative effects of George combining the two discrete experiences of his relationship with his father and with his son echoed our earlier academic discussions about photosynthesis and alchemy. Photosynthesis is combining chlorophyll and light to get energy while alchemy is combining different metals and an artisan to make gold. Both can be viewed as metaphors for *psychological transformation:* the combining of discrete experiences to catalyze a higher level of being, of awareness, of integration.

A month later, father and son sauntered into my office with a levity that was apparent. Larry reported that he had learned more about his dad's childhood that he hadn't before shared with anyone—stories about his friendships, first dates, goals, and fears. Larry and his wife had also invited his dad and mom to their home for what they touted would be "a healthy, gourmet dinner." The main course was waffles with whipped cream and ice cream. George kept saying what a wonderful time he had.

***

I still see George when he visits Boston, usually once a year. Like his presentation on financial planning, exercise, and ecology at the hearing loss conference where we had originally met, our discussions seldom have to do with hearing loss. Once in a while, he catches me up on the latest technological advances in assistive listening devices. Recently he told me that his son flat-out insisted on scheduling an appointment with an audiologist for a hearing aid evaluation; and "I dared not say no." Larry had also bought him a new television with a more advanced audio system and captioning.

We tend to talk about issues of connection, including his new-found intimacy with his children. George has come to more overtly cherish his emotional engagement with others. These needs had been thwarted by earlier patterns of alienation with his parents and were then exacerbated by his progressive hearing loss. Recently, George told me in passing that his sex life had improved as "my wife says I'm easier to be with."

Surprisingly, we also often talk about God. As he was a trained biologist, I had naively assumed that he would have scoffed at anything so nonempirical or scientific. Not so. His spirituality became clear as he described God as the grand operating system that regulates biological processes from microorganisms to plants to animals to humans: "The grand ecosystem is a carefully balanced organism with a wisdom whose voice I always strain to hear!"

George helped me understand a basic tenet of Jungian psychology: that the greater part of the soul is outside the body. In the words of psychologist James Hillman, "The world comes with shapes, colors, atmospheres, textures—a display of self-presenting forms. Things speak and announce themselves, bear witness to their presence... *Our imaginative recognition, the childlike act of imagining the world, animates the world and returns it to soul.*[4]

Until I met George, I had never heard trees and plants talk to me. I don't announce this revelation to many people, for fear it will be misunderstood. But I once announced it to George. He smiled, put his arm on my shoulder, and said, "It's okay, Mike. They talk to me, too."

Notes

1. Steinbeck, J. (1980). *Travels with Charley: In search of America.* New York: Viking Penguin.

2. Groopman, J. (1997). *The measure of our days: A spiritual exploration of illness.* New York: Penguin Books.

3. Pittman, F. (1990). The masculine mystique. *Family therapy networker,* May/June, 40–52.

4. Hillman, J. (1992). *The thought of the heart and soul of the world.* Dallas, TX: Spring Publications.

CHAPTER 6

Vicarious Hearing Loss: A Spouse's Tale

"I lost my hearing, then I lost my wife!" Mark lamented.

"Please say more," I said.

"I know she cares and is trying to help. But she doesn't get it! It seems that all she does is give me never-ending advice: 'Are your hearing aids working? Go to this doctor, to that doctor. You're better off than so-and-so—count your blessings. It'll get better. Relax. It's somehow part of God's plan. Get out and do something. Exercise more. Do yoga. Play golf. Get professional help.'"

"Why do you think she does this?" I asked.

"As I said, it's out of love; it's her way of helping."

"It also sounds like she, too, is desperate," I conjectured. "Both of you probably feel like you're losing each other."

Mark nodded his head sadly. Now 48 years old with two children, a solid marriage of over 20 years, and what should have been the height of his career as a high-level manager, his world had caved in. Two years ago, he woke up one morning with no hearing in one ear; then over the next several days, the hearing in his other ear began to fluctuate. After repeated visits to internists, otolaryngologists, neurologists, immunologists, radiologists, audiologists, and after countless tests, the diagnosis has remained "cause unknown." "Perhaps a virus, a rare immunological disorder, undetectable neurologic degeneration..." The doctors' long list of diagnostic possibilities was nothing compared to the list of potential life-threatening illnesses that plagued Mark during his darkest moments.

Mark felt assaulted not only by his loss of hearing and fear of death but also by "the cold indifference of the medical profession." After repeated assurances that "the doctor will definitely call you back before...", Mark knew he would receive no call-backs. They didn't seem to care. In many ways, he felt betrayed more by the physicians than by his ears.

I wondered though why he also felt betrayed by his wife. He referred to a widening chasm that separated them, leaving him feeling increasingly estranged from her and desperately alone. But he had never questioned her commitment to their marriage, continually emphasized that "she's always there for me" and realized, in his own words, "that she tries to help me out of love."

Mark himself was keenly aware of the paradox. "I know it doesn't make sense: She's there but not there. I shouldn't feel this way after all she's done. After all she continues to do for me."

"Let's figure it out," I responded. "What ways has she *not* been there for you while being there?"

He needed no time to respond. "She doesn't realize what this is like for me."

"This?" I asked.

"The roller coaster I've been on."

A metaphor for some very complicated feelings, I thought. I motioned for him to continue.

"I'm terrified and all alone—consumed by a *huge, vacuous, black hole.*"

"And what do you need from your wife?"

"For her to be on the roller coaster with me, at my side."

Mark's metaphors echoed a main tenet of object relations theory: namely, that one's sense of self cannot exist as a complete, cohesive structure—that is, cannot generate an experience of well being—

apart from nurturing responses from other key persons. Without deep connections with significant others, we shrivel up and disappear into "huge black holes."

The deep connection that Mark so desperately needed with Carolyn was to experience a sense of *merger*, a complete loss of boundaries and separateness. It is a universal need. Many people achieve this sense of merger during the height of sexual passion, others during intimate conversation. "He thinks my thoughts, completes my sentences." Cherished pets are often vehicles for this experience. Some achieve merger during a spiritual practice or meditation. Others resort to drug use, for example with hallucinogens that cause the boundaries of self and other to temporarily collapse. But with or without drugs, the merger experience is transitory, and remains elusive. Nevertheless, it is among the most sought-after of all human experiences, frequently leading one to sacrifice family ties, huge sums of money—even one's own life.

Mark looked uncomfortable after disclosing his hope for his wife's company on his private roller coaster, and quickly added, "I don't really mean I want her to suffer with me; I'm not that selfish. I wouldn't wish that on anybody!"

I invited him to say more.

"It's very simple," he replied softly. "I just want her to understand how I feel."

Simple words, I thought, for a complex array of thoughts and feelings. Human beings have struggled with that wish since the beginning and undoubtedly will continue to do so forever.

I suggested to Mark that we invite his wife to our next meeting, both so he could share with her his private terror and so that she could share hers with him. He took my next available appointment. He would also bring a portable FM system with a microphone that we could pass around to make sure he understood the three-way conversation. "With just you, it's easy," he said. "But with three people, I'm liable to miss things."

Carolyn was everything I expected: compassionate, articulate, and capable. She also acted in deference to Mark. Upon entering my office, she waited until he chose his preferred seat; only then did she take a seat adjacent to him. Although a particular seating arrangement often means absolutely nothing—and, in fact, its overinterpretation is a favorite past-time of neophyte therapists—in this case, it was diagnostic of their relationship: his needs were primary. After returning my handshake and agreeing that "it's nice to meet you, too," she was sure to add, "I'm very grateful to you for helping my husband."

"Both of you have gone through hell," I replied. I attempted to immediately expand the locus of "hell" to encompass not just Mark, but also Carolyn. I was tempted to use Mark's metaphors of a roller coaster and black hole, but most likely they would not be shared by Carolyn. Hell was probably inclusive enough.

"You can say that again," Carolyn sighed. "I'm very worried about him." Another sigh.

In this manner, she had acknowledged her own familiarity with hell, but shifted the focus back to him, deeming his pain as worse. It would be necessary to begin with her view of what is important. Later, I would attempt to expand the focus.

"What are you most worried about?" I asked.

"Mark is a good, good man. I couldn't have wished for a better husband or father for our children. He helps the whole world, except himself. And now, after going to a slew of doctors, nobody can tell us what's causing his hearing loss. He's having trouble sleeping, he doesn't find pleasure in much of anything, he's feeling hopeless and depressed, he's having trouble working. I'm really scared. What will they find next?"

"Who's 'they'?" I asked.

"All the goddamn doctors who haven't figured out what's going on, why this is happening. It absolutely kills me to see him in this much pain."

In describing Mark, it seemed that Carolyn had provided me with the easy opening to her own that I was hoping for. "I'm sure it does kill you to see him this way," I said. "Can you tell me what that's like for you?"

"Dr. Harvey, Mark's the one who needs the most help. I'm okay." Her voice showed mild irritation.

Her door slammed shut. Or maybe the opening was a false one or more obscure than I had thought. In order to decide between these two possibilities, I opted to push the issue a bit.

"What Mark has gone through doesn't affect you?" I asked, admittedly more provocatively than intended. Perhaps, I was being overzealous and intervening prematurely.

"Of course it has. But it has affected him a lot more; it happened, after all, *to him.*"

"I agree. He's sustained a direct hearing loss; but you've sustained a *vicarious* hearing loss?"

"Huh?" came her predictable reply.

"It's a strange thing," I responded, deliberately slowly, looking straight into her eyes. *"My daughter was stung by a bee the other day. I swear it hurt me more than her."*

Carolyn paused, then nodded and looked to the floor. She then returned my gaze. I had struck a nerve.

"For parents, our vicarious bee stings hurt more than the direct kind that sting our kids. There's nothing worse than seeing somebody we love in so much pain. And even more frustrating, our vicarious bee stings can't be treated with rubbing alcohol, Benadryl, or whatever. We just kind of sit with it, wishing we could make it better. But we can't."

What I had said released a torrent of repressed tears; then her face began to spasm and another layer of protective composure gave way to audible sobbing. Her torment suddenly became fully visible to Mark and I. After a few moments, I invited her to share what she was feeling.

This time her answer came from deep within, apparently without being filtered through her head. She cried, "I can't make it go away! I can't make it better!" She cried more, falling deeper into her previously hidden pit of despair. "I can't make it go away; I can't make it better." She poured out this phrase again and again, soon in a whisper. It seemed that she had uttered these phrases many times, but nobody had heard them.

Carolyn then apologized.

"For what?" I asked. Mark, who was at the edge of his seat, echoed with "Please don't apologize. It's okay, sweetheart. I know how hard this is for you."

"I'm sorry, Mark. I'm so sorry." More tears.

"What are you sorry for, sweetie?" Mark pleaded.

"It's been so hard for you. I don't want to make it worse."

At this point, I interjected to Carolyn, "'After all he's been through, what right do I have to have feelings?'"

"Yeah, something like that," came her instant response. She tried to squelch her tears.

"Feelings are something we have, whether or not we have a right to them."

"It's something I try not to think about," Carolyn admitted. "I'm just happy he's alive; I'm grateful when there's even a minute hope of improvement; I admire his courage, his strength, how he keeps on going—"

"Excuse me," I broke in, "but I was asking—"

"—me how I feel," she interrupted. "I know. Okay, okay! It's hard for me, too." A five-word preview of her own suffering, I thought. Carolyn then glanced at Mark, perhaps for fear that she had done something wrong, maybe that she had, even then, just hurt him in some way. Her expression became distant and she clammed up. I sensed that she, too, desperately needed the kind of merger experience that Mark needed from her. Except that she did not feel deserving of it.

Therefore, at this juncture, I calmly said to Carolyn, "You know, you may be afraid of hurting him by putting words to your feelings. We could ask him to leave the room, but I'm willing to bet you that he already knows what you'll say. But saying how you feel will, in the long run, help him hurt less; and, by the way, will help you, too." I thought of Nietzsche who said that "silence is poison." I asked Mark to remain seated in front of Carolyn but at a 45-degree angle so she would not predominately see his face. We took some time to test his FM system to ensure that he would continue to be able to understand both of us.

For several moments, we sat in silence. Mark tried to persuade her to begin, but I motioned him to stop. I sensed that Carolyn needed the stillness and silence of these moments to allow her long-stifled torment to rise to the surface and fully express itself. Finally she began. "Yes, it's been awful. And I've been so lonely throughout all of this. I don't know what to do. Nobody understands how cut off I feel from everyone, even from my husband whom I love more than I can ever say. I need him desperately. But he has enough to deal with without hearing about my pain." She fell silent.

"So you feel guilty adding to his burden?"

She nodded her head in shame.

My query was, in large part, prompted by Professor David Luterman's book, *In the Shadows: Living and Coping with a Loved One's Chronic Illness.* It is about his own experiences being married to a wife who has multiple sclerosis.[1] As a nondisabled spouse, he, too, often remained in the shadows, feeling an almost inexplicable loneliness. As Luterman put it,

> It is the rare individual who looks at me and asks me how I am doing; almost everyone wants to know, and it's understandable, how my wife is. Occasionally though, I need some attention. When I do ask for attention, it is always tinged with guilt as though I do not have the right to complain. People almost always look at the person in the wheelchair, seldom at the person pushing it.[2] (p. xvii)

"I can tell when she's upset because she goes to the basement and watches TV," Mark volunteered.

"And do you go to the basement with her?"

"Not usually," he admitted. "I figure she needs space from me."

"Sometimes that's probably true, but there seems to be too much space," I observed.

"But sometimes, she gets irritable and curt with me for no reason, as if I can do nothing right." Now Mark had an edge to his voice, and I got a further glimpse of the chasm between them.

I decided to follow a hunch. Turning again to Carolyn, I asked, "Does it also feel to you like the person you would most like to share your pain with is the cause of it?"

Now she abruptly arched back in her seat and remained motionless for several seconds. Then she made her confession, "Yeah, sometimes when Mark's hearing loss hits rock bottom, I silently scream 'Why did you do this to me?'" Her jaw tightened and she looked away.

"This?" I asked.

"I sometimes get very angry with him for no clear reason," she again admitted after taking a breath. "Sometimes just watching him makes me feel terrified and helpless. And then I feel so alone. I think to myself why does he make me so bloody scared? Why does he make me so lonely? Why does he put me on that goddamn roller coaster with him?" she grimaced. But then she retreated into her seat and her face showed despair. After her inadvertent release of anger, her valve abruptly closed and she began crying again.

"It's complicated," I said to Carolyn. "As you know—at least intellectually—Mark isn't 'doing this' to you: making you scared and lonely. But on an emotional, gut level, it must be sometimes hard to hold on to this. Normal human emotions, like anger, seldom follow the laws of reason."

"I'm sorry," she cried again looking desperately toward her husband. "The last thing you need is for me to get angry."

Carolyn vacillated between feeling terror, anger/rage, and guilt. Of course, she knew that the responsible culprit was whatever caused his hearing loss, not Mark per se. But her responses were not unusual. Generally, the loneliness that the "shadow spouse" experiences frequently gets eclipsed by anger, for it is more empowering than loneliness. But, in their particular case, since the cause of Mark's condition was obscure, vague, faceless, without prognosis, it was spared her wrath. Inevitably, Mark himself became the lightning rod.

Ironically, both found themselves feeling abandoned by the other. A vicious cycle: Mark feels traumatized; Carolyn feels Mark's trauma and tries to help; Mark's trauma worsens; Carolyn feels scared, overwhelmed, angry, and isolated; out of self-preservation and guilt, she disengages emotionally and acts upbeat in front of Mark; he feels scared, overwhelmed, angry, and isolated; out of self-preservation and guilt, he also disengages emotionally and acts upbeat in front of Carolyn; Mark again feels traumatized, etc.

I felt a deep sense of compassion for Carolyn, as well as for Mark who was taking in all of what she finally had voiced openly. He had understood every word. I asked him whether any of what she said was a surprise to him.

"No, not at all!" he replied with tears of his own. "But honey," he continued. "You don't have to get so scared and lonely. Please don't."

"I shouldn't feel lonely or scared?" she abruptly shot back, now sarcastically and with incredulousness. More of her anger was revealed.

"It makes me feel awful to see you suffer so much," Mark defended himself.

Now I jumped in. "Carolyn, one doesn't need to be a rocket scientist to figure out why you would feel scared, lonely, angry, desperate, depressed—"

"You got that right," she agreed, now obviously feeling validated. I was in danger, however, of fostering collusion against Mark.

"But Mark does have a point," I quickly interjected. "I wonder if there are other experiences or losses that you've had—that you've brought to the relationship—that somehow cause you to react with *more* fear, *more* loneliness, *more* anger than you otherwise would've."

Initially Carolyn looked as if she would retaliate. But then she sat still and had no difficulty answering my question; her memory search took less than a second. "My father was diagnosed with cancer when I was 13 years old."

I felt my body stiffen, knowing what was to come.

"And what happened?" I had to ask.

Carolyn whispered something unintelligible and looked down. Mark then supplied the answer. "He died a horrible death."

We fell silent. They would tell me later that her father's fatal illness began with undiagnosable mild pain, localized to his stomach. Thus, Carolyn naturally filled in the blanks of Mark's "etiology of hearing loss unknown" condition—so far localized to his ears—with traumatic memories of her father's horrible death.

"It must terrify you to see Mark this way," I finally said.

She nodded her head.

Mark then moved his seat closer to his wife, correctly sensing that Carolyn was scared that he, too, would die. I had a sense of what he must have been feeling. After all, didn't he—only two weeks ago—tell me that he wished for Carolyn to be on the roller coaster with him at his side? Although his merger needs were quite legitimate, as were Carolyn's, they were likely to produce guilt. Be careful what you wish for, I thought. Mark confirmed my hunch by meekly saying to Carolyn, "I'm sorry you're scared and lonely. It's my fault."

"Don't be silly, sweetheart, it's not your fault," Carolyn assured him, again becoming the unconditionally supportive wife.

"You're right," I replied. "It's a complicated thing," I emphasized, facing Carolyn. "On the one hand, Mark doesn't want you to feel scared and lonely on a roller coaster with him; but, on the other hand, he very much does. It's not that he's selfish, mean, or sadistic. It's a normal and understandable wish." I said to both of them what a gift it is to have a partner with whom to share your soul.

"And Carolyn, you've very bravely *begun* to share with us some of what you desperately need Mark to understand, what feelings you also wish him to feel with you. So far, they've been from the outer edges of your soul, but it's a good start." It was both an acknowledgment of the important disclosures Carolyn had already made and an invitation for her to continue. She got both messages.

"Thanks," she said. "Yeah, whatever's happening to Mark does scare the shit out of me, but I've tried not to show it to him. But I know it hasn't worked; he knows me too well." For the first time, they both smiled. Mark nodded his head.

I asked Mark if he would like Carolyn to continue. Again, he nodded affirmatively.

Predictably, her smile gave way to fear. "It's a worst nightmare come true. I don't know what the future will bring, what other problems Mark will have." She paused, I imagined, to see if we were serious about bearing witness to her nightmare or whether we would give her some platitudes and change the subject. Mark and I remained silent.

"I don't know why this is happening," she finally continued. "I feel so helpless; I want to do something but I can't. And then I feel guilty sometimes for enjoying my life and doing things like listening to music. I sometimes feel so damn guilty because my hearing is alright. I've given up music; I cut my telephone conversations short. What right do I have to enjoy things when he's suffering so much? And look how God rewarded us for going to church every Sunday. No more of that!" she scowled.

"God doesn't follow you to the basement either?"

"God can you-know-what!" she retorted. Then her voice softened. "I don't know what this means for our children."

"What do you mean?" I asked.

"Will our kids get sick like Mark when they're his age? Maybe whatever's causing his hearing loss is genetic." Carolyn now showed more of her private terror. It encompassed far more than her husband's loss of hearing. She, too, had been consumed by a range of emotions and fears that she encoded with her own unique metaphors, the more painful ones probably having to do with cancer, I thought. The question had to be asked.

"Are you afraid, during your worst moments, that Mark will die?"

"Yes, I am." The valve between her mask and inner torment

opened, this time allowing her pain to come forth without restraint. Carolyn began heavy, gut-wrenching sobbing. Mark knelt beside her and hugged her, saying softly "It'll be alright, it'll be alright." But then he, too, began to cry, first with restraint and then also succumbing to despair. Several moments passed.

They remained clutched to each other, perhaps on a terrifying roller coaster ride, I thought. They seemed to lose awareness of my presence; and I, too, found myself in an altered, detached state. They began to rock each other back and forth in meditation-like, rhythmic motions. It became difficult to discern who initiated and who followed, and I began to imagine them as indistinguishable. This is what we had worked so hard to achieve. Only I wish it didn't hurt so much.

I continued to sit in awe as Mark and Carolyn rocked back and forth. It felt *mystical,* a kind of spiritual transcendence that was fueled by their obviously deep love for each other. It was Martin Luther King who said, "When I speak of love, I am speaking of that force which all the great religions have seen as the supreme unifying principle of life. Love is the key that unlocks the door which leads to ultimate reality."[3] It was happening right before my eyes.

Classical mystics speak of the expanding sense of self and the loss of personal consciousness; the achievement of "at-one-ment" with a divine essence. Rabbi Lawrence Kushner explained this spiritual principal another way. "You cannot become someone other than you are until you are willing, for just one moment, to allow yourself to become one whom you are *not.* That is, until you are willing to enter the Nothing. It is possibly the most effortless (and the most important) thing any of us can do."[4]

Although transformative, Mark and Carolyn's task of entering the abyss of "Nothing" was anything *but* effortless. Carolyn yearned for an empathic connection with Mark but fought it at every turn. And, as Mark later put it, "To get out of myself and then put myself in Carolyn's shoes—although it has saved me and our marriage—was more terrifying than even being on a roller coaster."

Their challenge encompassed more than empathizing with each other's pain. It was also to be vulnerable to the timeless void of surrendering who they were but not yet becoming the other; somewhere between I am not me but not you. Each of them had to go beyond and surrender their feelings without knowing what they would get in return. Merger is a terrifying, ecstatic, and sacred experience.

For Mark and Carolyn, it was also what they so desperately needed from each other. It would be only through this merger experience that they could evolve as individuals and support each other to better tolerate their respective ordeals. More importantly, however, Mark and Carolyn became privy to one of life's sacred lessons: that there can be redemption only in terror that is *shared*. Terror that remains private metastasizes to pollute first one's body and then one's soul.

***

A simple-sounding therapeutic exercise: For one-half hour, one spouse is instructed to talk about only him/herself; the other partner is to listen attentively, but to make no verbal responses whatsoever.[5] Mark and Carolyn had attempted to do that exercise around the time that I first met them.

Mark's metaphorical wish taken literally seemed safe enough for Carolyn to listen to attentively. A two-seat ride on a roller coaster with both of them securely strapped in. But in real life, there are no straps, no guaranteed safety. Similarly, for Mark to have empathetically understood Carolyn's experience of "vicarious hearing loss" would have meant confronting her worst fear for him—his death. Also a scary proposition, again without guaranteed safety.

As with many couples, with or without a hearing loss, Carolyn and Mark's needs, wishes, and frustrations were mirror images of the other. Although Mark was directly traumatized by the loss of hearing and other medical complications, Carolyn was vicariously traumatized. When one part of a family system is in pain, every part is affected.

However, both of them, until recently, had deemed only *his* direct trauma needs and feelings worthy of attention. The needs of "shadow spouses" are ignored—often by others, often by themselves. Recall Carolyn's own words. "Dr. Harvey, Mark's the one who needs the most help. I'm okay."

We met regularly on a weekly basis for about three months, working hard to disrupt that cycle that left both feeling abandoned by the other. Our work together consisted of the same amazing, but not surprising, milestones that all couples face: how to support each other; how to achieve that magical, sacred state of merger with the other, and at the same time, come to terms with feeling betrayed by its elusiveness and finiteness. Like other such experiences, it tends to happen when we least expect it.

Mark's hearing continued to fluctuate for reasons unknown. Similarly, Carolyn's optimism and confidence continued to fluctuate. But they were no longer alone.

Notes

1. Luterman, D. (1995). *In the shadows: Living and coping with a loved one's chronic illness.* Bedford, MA: Jade Press.
2. Luterman, D. (1995). *In the shadows: Living and coping with a loved one's chronic illness.* Bedford, MA: Jade Press.
3. King, M. L. (1967). *Where do we go from here: Chaos of community.*
4. Kushner, L. (1981). *The river of light: Spirituality, Judaism, consciousness.* Woodstock, VT: Jewish Lights.
5. Scarf, M. (1987). *Intimate partners.* New York: Ballantine Books.

CHAPTER 7

Beyond the Tug-of-War

Jim and Debbie Harris were a pleasant, middle-class, deaf couple who had a 2-year-old hearing son whom they unfortunately brought to the meeting. He had mastered the art of locomotion and vocalization and was locomoting and vocalizing all over my office. Within minutes, the Legos were thrown all over my floor, the box of Kleenex was gutted, and everyone in the adjoining office was complaining about the racket.

This unexpected distraction added to my already mild anxiety about meeting them. When initially meeting deaf couples whose primary language is American Sign Language, I typically feel a little anxious about whether we will be able to easily understand each other. As a hearing person, ASL is not my native language. Thankfully, it turned out that communication was not a problem. Both Jim and Debbie signed American Sign Language beautifully; and they reported that they understood my ASL as well.

Jim defined himself as having a profound hearing loss, which had been progressive since early adolescence. He wore hearing aids and kept up-to-date on the latest technological developments in audiology. He would jump at the chance to take a magic pill to regain his hearing, and was considering getting a cochlear implant. Debbie, however, defined herself as culturally Deaf. She was born with a profound hearing loss and had attended a school for the Deaf until her graduation. She wanted no part of the hearing world, even if she could "become one of them." She did not define herself as disabled as did Jim; she defined herself as part of the Deaf community. Debbie went to Association of Late Deafened Adults (ALDA) or Self-Help for the Hard-of-Hearing (SHHH) conventions with Jim at his request and Jim went to National Association of the Deaf (NAD) conventions with Debbie at her request.

I often experience another distraction when meeting Deaf clients for the first time: my need to take notes typically wins over focusing solely on our discussion. Unlike with hearing clients when it is possible to talk, listen, and write at the same time, I needed to frequently interrupt the dialogue with Jim and Debbie to jot down notes. While I typically have a pretty good memory for stories and demographic facts, I first need a context, a cognitive container, to put them in. So the better part of our initial meeting was spent constructing a genogram (see Figure 1), a favorite container of sorts among family therapists to keep track of who's who.

Figure 1.

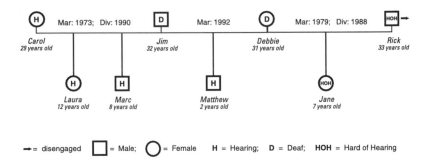

Jim and Debbie met at a Deaf community function six years prior, several months after Jim had been separated from his hearing wife and one year after Debbie had been divorced from her Deaf husband. They married three years later.

"No, Matthew," Jim yelled. "You can't touch the doctor's desk. It's not yours. Now come over here and play with your Legos!"

"Thanks," I responded. (I had important papers on my desk.) Back to the genogram.

Jim has two hearing children from his previous marriage, 12-year-old Laura and 8-year-old Marc, who he sees every other weekend and some weeknights.

"Matthew, come here! We told you..." This time Debbie retrieved him.

"Boy, he's a handful," I observed with mock calmness and flexibility. They nodded their heads. Back to the genogram.

Debbie has a hard-of-hearing child from her previous marriage, 7-year-old Jane, of whom she has full custody. Jane's father had moved out of state.

"Matthew, come here!" Down went my plant and dirt went all over my rug. Matthew was made to sit down between his parents. Back to the genogram.

Jane's father sees her only sporadically. Jim and Debbie have a 2-year-old son, Matthew, who is hearing. I didn't need a genogram to know that.

Luckily, it was almost time to end our first meeting. Before we stopped, however, I needed to ask them why they came (except for their kid to destroy my office, I thought).

Jim responded that they were having problems with Laura, his 12-year-old, hearing daughter from his previous marriage.

"What problems?" I asked.

"She complains about coming over all the time and when she finally does, she throws temper tantrums and blockades herself in her bedroom. And in school she's absent a lot and her grades are going down."

"Uh-huh. I see. Okay, let's arrange another meeting. Could we also invite Laura and Marc? And uh, it uh, may be a lot faster if you can get a babysitter for this guy," I smiled.

"Yeah," Debbie agreed. "We were going to leave him at the sitter today, but she canceled at the last minute."

"Cute kid," I lied.

We bid goodbye. In reviewing our first meeting, I marveled at the immense challenges of forming postdivorce families, often called blended, reconstituted, or step-families. As a first marriage signifies the joining of two families, a second marriage involves the inter-weaving of three, four, or more families, whose previous family life cycle course has been disrupted by death or divorce. At this writing, at least 35% of children can expect to live with a stepparent for some time before the age of 18.[1]

Laura's apparent difficulty in engaging with a new family config-uration is certainly not unusual. A renewed sense of belonging fre-quently takes three to five years to develop—longer if the children are adolescents. Often children feel abandoned by the noncustodial parent. Clashes between stepparents and stepchildren are common, as children often feel a rigid loyalty to their biological parents. Step-parents—predictably less emotionally attached to their spouse's chil-dren—may feel displaced and exploited during the children's visits. Stepparents may have to deal with the fact that their spouse's copar-enting partnership is conducted more with the ex-spouse than with him or her. Also, because the parent–child bond predates the mari-tal bond, stepparents may feel insecure and unwittingly compete with their stepchildren for primacy with their spouse, as if the rela-tionships were on the same level.

Although blended families offer many profound, invaluable re-wards for all of their members, they don't just smoothly *blend* to-gether as the name implies. There are countless challenges and land mines, even without deafness-related communication issues added to the mix. The Harris family was no exception.

A week later, I entered my waiting room to greet the family. First

I noticed who thankfully was *not* there: Matthew. There is a God after all, I thought. I made eye contact with Jim and Debbie who smiled back, perhaps reading my thoughts. Then I introduced myself in sim-comma to Jim's children, Laura and Marc. They were good looking kids. Eight-year-old Marc looked shy and soft-spoken, maybe even a bit scared. Twelve-year-old Laura had a more expressive and assertive expression that seemed to say, "I have better things to do than be here for a boring meeting but I was forced to come so I'll be polite and put up with it but don't expect me to have fun or benefit in any way so let's get this over with so I can go home and call my friends."

Out of both of their mouths, however, came only "It's nice to meet you, too." But nothing "came out" of their hands—they were not signing. I realized that I had neglected to ask Jim and Debbie earlier whether the kids were competent in a signed language. I bookmarked that observation in my head and beckoned the four of them into my office.

Jim began the meeting with essentially a summary of his concerns about Laura that he had told me a week ago. He used sim-comm with good vocal intelligibility.[a]

Laura responded to her father with only her voice. "Get off my back!" she yelled.

Debbie said to Jim in ASL (naturally without voice) that she didn't understand what Laura said. Jim then interpreted Laura's statement in ASL for Debbie.

"I do good in school, Daddy." Marc jumped in, also with only his voice.

"Shut up you goody-two-shoes," Laura yelled to her brother.

"You shut up yourself," Marc said.

They argued back and forth. I couldn't tell whether Jim was able to effectively speech read their oral ping-ponging and whether he

---

a. Simultaneous communication, often abbreviated as "sim-comm," is the use of
    visually coded English or Pidgin Sign English while vocalizing English words.

understood the meanings of their English idioms, "Get off my back!" and "goody-two-shoes" although, given that the onset of his hearing loss was late adolescence, his English would probably be solid. I sensed that Debbie, their stepmother, was completely lost in the conversation.

A familiar beginning. When meeting a nonsigning family in which there is a signing Deaf member, the immediate challenge is to establish the communication logistics of the session. However, to do that, one needs to communicate; and typically someone is initially left out of the loop. Perhaps the cleanest beginning would have been for me to sequentially voice then sign, or vice versa. However, I was concerned about prematurely calling too much attention to what appeared to be a communication chasm between Jim and Debbie and the kids. I did not want them to perceive me as too confrontive or judgmental. Furthermore, at least in the meeting with his children present, Jim chose to sim-comm. Therefore, at least for now, I, too, chose to use Pidgin Sign English while vocalizing.

For every logistic decision that the therapist makes about communication, there are therapeutic advantages and compromises.[2] One advantage of the communication option of simultaneous communication is that it is initially a bit less awkward and confronting to hearing, nonsigning family members than if the therapist signs without voice. Furthermore, assuming that English is linguistically accessible to the deaf member, the therapist can more easily convey a message to the deaf member while simultaneously addressing a hearing member.

A disadvantage of this option, however, has to do with clarity of communication. English is often not a culturally Deaf member's primary mode of communication. (Pidgin Signed English was largely accessible for Jim but totally inaccessible for Debbie whose primary language was American Sign Language.) Second, it is clearer to either sign *or* use voice; both modes of communication suffer when done simultaneously.[3] Finally, sim-comm does not adequately demonstrate the sophistication and beauty of American Sign Language in its own right.

Jim told me in sim-comm that Laura and Marc had never "wanted to sign as it was too hard." Laura sighed and looked away. Marc looked a bit sad.

"Signing is very hard for us hearing people," I replied to Jim in sim-comm. "It's very hard," my eyes met Laura's, "But what a shame!"

"Shame about what?" Laura scowled.

I got her interest. In sim-comm, I responded to her that "You and your father probably have a lot of things that you want to say to each other, but you have different ways of communicating. And I bet you're also missing a lot of what comes from your stepmother; and she misses what comes from you."

Jim and Debbie nodded, which I took to mean that they understood at least a chunk of what I was saying. I would check that out later.

"He understands me okay," Laura assured me.

"How often do you test your assumption?" I asked.

"What do you mean?"

"Well, for starters, how often do you see each other?"

"On weekends every two weeks usually."

I thought to myself that those roughly four days per month don't add up to a lot of time, particularly since Laura apparently often spent much of her time in the bedroom. I wondered why. What hidden or not-so-hidden alliances or coalitions existed between Laura and her hearing mother that excluded Jim and Debbie.

"Does your mom know sign language?" I asked Laura in sim-comm.

"Not really," came her oral reply.

I asked for confirmation from Jim in ASL.

Jim, in turn, responded in ASL. "My ex-wife was never really interested in learning sign language. When we were married, she signed a little but not much. That was a big reason why we got divorced." Debbie perked up, now finally able to easily understand what was being discussed.

Now Laura looked a bit thrown off guard, perhaps not knowing what to make of me and her father signing without our voices. As much as her initial countenance reflected her not wanting to be here, she apparently didn't enjoy being conversationally excluded. That is an experience deaf people know well.

"Would you interpret what you said for Laura?" I asked Jim, now in sim-comm.

"Your mother didn't know much sign language," Jim told his daughter.

I accepted Jim's truncated interpretation. "Aren't you just a wee bit curious why not?" I asked Laura.

"Why not what?" she responded.

"Why a deaf and a hearing person would be married to each other for 17 years and not use the same language? You know, if a Chinese person married a Spanish person, after a while wouldn't you think that they would agree to speak one language or the other? How would they watch TV? What newspaper would they buy? How would they order take-out? How would they know what to get each other for their birthdays? How would they decide who's using the bathroom before—"

"My dad lipreads," Laura finally interjected.

"How effective do you think lipreading is?"

"He lipreads good," she said confidently.

"Good enough to understand everything that you want to say to him?" I asked.

"Yeah," came her terse reply. Then she shot a look of loathing at her father.

I turned to her and said, "Or maybe you don't have a lot to say to your dad. Maybe you're angry at him? Maybe you feel hurt?, I don't know—you tell me."

"I talk to him enough; and I understand his voice. But it's boring over at his house," Laura's complained. "Plus Matthew's a pain in the butt."

"Yeah, he's a real handful," I said. For an instant, we made empathic eye contact. I continued, "It must be boring if you can't understand your stepmother at all and your dad has trouble understanding you." My statement caused Laura to look down in disgust. I had gone too far too soon. It was time to try a different, less provocative approach.

"Laura, what do you like to do when you're over at your house with your mother?"

"Hang out."

"Hang out how?"

"Just hang out."

"I mean do you hang from a rope, from the curtains, from the chandelier?" I joked. Maybe humor would facilitate this adult–adolescent interchange.

"I mean hang out. You know, hang out!" She wasn't amused.

Humor wouldn't work. "Okay, okay. I get it," I said. "Do you also hang out with your dad and stepmom?"

"It's boring over there, I just told you that!" she frowned.

"It's not boring. I have fun!" Marc interjected.

"Ah. You have fun but Laura doesn't. Why do you think your sister doesn't have fun?" I asked Marc.

"They sign all the time there," he responded.

"Marc's right," Jim jumped in. "I think a lot of our problems are related to communication."

"That seems to be a piece of the problem," I agreed.

My mind was on a different track, however. The data: Two hearing kids grow up with a deaf dad and hearing mom; deaf dad signs, hearing mom doesn't sign and kids don't sign; parents get divorced; hearing kids visit deaf dad infrequently; and at least one is oppositional to him. The hypotheses: (1) an alliance of hearing mom and hearing children that excludes deaf dad/stepmom and (2) perhaps a coalition of the hearies against the deafies, with at least subtle degradation.

I found myself imagining Laura as a victim of a tug-of-war

between her biological parents—a conflict of loyalties that unfortunately often comes with divorce. But in Laura's case, this dynamic had an additional twist, for it involved a tension between hearing and deaf loyalties. Her hearing mother had "pulled in" Laura harder than had her deaf father, as evidenced by Laura's disengagement with her father and minimal, if any, interest or knowledge of sign language.

However, as Marc and his dad correctly noted, communication was certainly a huge piece of the problem. (It always impresses me how young kids have the knack for blurting out the truth unabashedly). Many, if not all, couples and families come in complaining about "communication problems." Most of the time, *hearing* people mean that they cannot mind-read each other or that they fight too much. However, when deaf-member families acknowledge themselves as having "communication problems," they typically mean not just mind-reading and negotiating breakdowns, but also inadequate language exchange. In this case, Jim and Debbie were frequently unable to understand fully what the hearing kids were saying orally; and the hearing kids often had trouble understanding Debbie and Jim.

If only the solution were as simple as "You should take sign language classes." It's not that simple. The challenge is to untangle "generic" dysfunctional patterns from those specific to language barriers.

I would begin with Debbie, who had displayed a blank expression for the last half-hour. Laura and Marc's oral conversation had been completely inaccessible to her, while Jim's and my English-based signing were largely inaccessible. I wanted to acknowledge and support Debbie for what undoubtedly had to be her feelings of disconnection or alienation with respect to our discussion and second, to begin "untangling" those linguistic barriers from whatever affections or animosities there may have been between Debbie and the kids.

In ASL, Debbie confirmed that she had no idea of what everyone had been talking about. She looked disheartened, as did Jim. But then she gave a surprising response. She asked, "Why don't we get an interpreter?"

Jim sim-commed "An interpreter!"

The kids voiced "An interpreter!"

Suddenly our therapeutic discourse became a chorus. I asked Debbie to say more.

In ASL, she gave her reply. "An interpreter would help me understand what Laura and Marc are saying and would help them understand me. Jim would also not have to work so hard lipreading, and I know he also misses a lot and feels bad about that." Jim then orally interpreted Debbie's analysis for the kids.

Perhaps anticipating Laura and Marc's concerns, Jim immediately explained that "like a therapist, an interpreter also keeps everything private." It seemed that Jim, following his initial surprise, supported Debbie's idea.

Predictably, Marc responded with "Neat!" Also predictably, Laura said nothing.

To Laura, I asked, "Who would you rather have here, an interpreter or Matthew?"

"An interpreter!" she immediately proclaimed. This time, she smiled.

Over the years, I have done a lot of thinking about the benefits of including an interpreter in family therapy for nonsigning families in which the deaf member's primary language is a signed language.[4] Obviously, an interpreter facilitates language exchange. The interpreter interprets voice to sign so the deaf member can understand others' vocal communications, and interprets sign to voice so the hearing members can understand the deaf member's signed communications. Although a therapist may be fluent in manual communication and perhaps may even be certified as an interpreter, it is usually neither feasible nor therapeutically prudent to interpret while simultaneously providing treatment. Both are discrepant, complex, and energy-consuming tasks.

The potential benefits of an interpreter, however, go far beyond facilitating language exchange. The interpreter becomes a beacon of sorts, an unambiguous *symbol of deaf empowerment,* and irrefutable evidence that the deaf member is competent. The inclusion of an interpreter is a systemic intervention for upsetting the power balance in a family system (or for that matter, in any system) in which the integrity and, in fact, humanity of the deaf member have been suppressed. For example, the language barrier between Debbie and Jim's children had metaphorically reduced her presence to that of a two-dimensional, cardboard prop.

Debbie listed her preferred interpreters, all of whom had experience working in family therapy and mental health settings. I offered to set up the logistics. We made an appointment for three weeks. I also asked that Jane, Debbie's 7-year-old, hard-of-hearing daughter, also attend the meeting. I was curious about what influence she would have on Debbie's hopefully emerging presence and on the rest of the family. Jane's appearance would also provide an opportunity to forge beginning alliances among the three siblings.

Three weeks later, Allison, the interpreter, and I met a few minutes before the meeting in order to review language considerations and provide her with a rough sketch of my treatment goals. This is my standard procedure. Typically, I schedule a presession meeting with an interpreter; then the therapy session takes place; and then the family leaves while the interpreter remains for a postsession meeting. Such pre- and postsession meetings are necessary for effective therapist-interpreter teamwork to occur.[5-7]

I had worked with Allison many times before. Our presession lasted less than five minutes. We went over the rough goals of the meeting and the communication logistics: I would sign for myself with the deaf family members and voice for the hearing members, while Allison would voice and sign interpret, respectively. She would also interpret intrafamilial communication.

It was time for the session. Allison and I greeted the family and escorted them into the office. I motioned for the family members to choose their seats; then I asked Jim and Debbie to determine where Allison should sit. I took the remaining seat. Everybody seemed a bit anxious with the two newcomers: the interpreter and Jane. I therefore took the lead and asked Allison to explain issues of confidentiality. She outlined the relevant RID (Registry of Interpreters for the Deaf) Code of Ethics, first in sim-comm and then in ASL. Everyone seemed satisfied.

Then I acknowledged Jane. She looked her age of seven years, dressed in red shorts and a Rug Rats T-shirt. From doing the genogram, I had learned that she was born with a moderate hearing loss, cause unknown. Her then 26-year-old father—also hard-of-hearing—was an alcoholic and left Debbie and Jane for another woman soon after Jane was born.

I asked Jane in sim-comm who her favorite Rug Rat's character was. (My then eight-year-old daughter had made me sit through countless episodes). Jane responded in sim-comm that she liked Angelica the best. Then Debbie, in ASL, asked her to explain why. Jane then gave an elaborate response to Debbie in beautiful ASL. (Allison voiced for Laura and Marc's benefit). Jane was bilingual in English and American Sign Language. She traversed comfortably in both the Deaf and the hearing worlds without being stuck in the limbo between two worlds, an experience that is familiar to many hard-of-hearing persons.[8]

It was time to elicit how Debbie viewed Jim's kids. In ASL with Allison voicing, I asked Debbie what she liked most about Laura and Marc. She articulately described Laura as a bright, very likable, creative, passionate, but confused adolescent. She described Marc as spunky, also very bright, but lonely.

"Please say more about Marc's loneliness," I said in ASL, while Allison voiced. So far Laura had been the lightening rod for family struggles while Marc had remained in the sidelines. It would be helpful to expand the focus a bit.

"I think he misses his dad; and he doesn't know what to make out of the bitterness between his parents. I think he wants to learn sign language but is afraid that his mom would be angry or disappointed."

Marc suddenly lost his sparkle and spunk and became quiet and sullen. In a soft voice, I asked him an either/or question, phrased appropriately to his age, "Do you think your mom would be happy or upset about you signing more?"

"Upset," came his instant reply. Then he thought for a moment and added, "Sometimes when I sign at home by mistake, she tells me not to."

"She does not!" Laura interjected.

"She does too!"

"She does not!" she yelled. Laura was obviously closely allied with her mother.

"She does too! Yesterday when..."

They bickered as they had done before in our meetings. It was clear that Laura was protecting her mother and Marc was the voice of truth. But this time, their bickering was accessible to both Jim and Debbie, whereas before they could only see it as meaningless, garbled lip movements.

Debbie waved her hands to stop their exchange and said in ASL (with Allison voicing), "You know, Laura, you can speak to your mother and sign with me. You don't have to choose; it doesn't have to be either/or."

Laura was looking in the opposite direction at Allison. "Excuse me," I interrupted. I asked Allison "Would you move over here in back of Laura?" I wanted to increase the eye contact between Debbie and Laura with the hope of increasing the likelihood of an alliance.

"Debbie, please continue," I said.

Now Debbie was able to make eye contact with Laura. "And the good part of us becoming better friends is that I would have someone to go shopping with. I know you like clothes shopping. I do, too. I absolutely *love* to go shopping downtown on Newbury Street! The stores, the boutiques... they're wonderful! But your father won't go with me; and even if he did, he complains too much and is boring to shop with. You know—*men!* I could use a young woman's advice."

"Mom hates Newbury Street, too," Marc chimed in. The function of his interruption wasn't clear. Was he jealous and meant to interrupt a potential intimacy between his sister and step-mother? Or was he playing matchmaker between his dad and mom?

Jim rightly ignored Marc's interruption and took Debbie's lead. "Maybe you can even get some clothes out of the deal."

"Both of you could bring Matthew!" I added.

"No way!" retorted Laura. We all laughed, knowing that in her own way, Laura had just accepted Debbie's offer.

While Debbie would not and *should not be* a substitute mother for Laura, she could be a good friend. I agree with the often-given advice to step-parents that they should try for and expect mutual courtesy, but not a stepchild's love. Then they may work out a relationship that supplements, but does not compete with, the special bond between the biological parent and child; a relationship that resembles a parent (or godparent), aunt or uncle, friend, or whatever model of mentor/nurturer that appeals to them. The love that may develop will be a by-product of this work, a miraculous surprise that cannot be purposely willed. In the right atmosphere, it grows on its own.

Now it was time to focus on Jane's relationship with her step-siblings. I asked Marc to tell me what he likes most about Jane. "After all, you're about the same age," I observed.

"She's not bad for a girl," Marc volunteered. "Mathew's a boy but I like Jane more."

"Do you hang out with her a lot?" I asked.

"We don't 'hang out.' That's what Laura does; I don't do that. We play on the computer instead."

"I see. I'll remember that from now on. Does she sign with you at all?" I wondered whether the hearing–deaf tug-of-war extended to Marc and Jane.

"Yeah," Marc replied. "She's taught me some neat signs."

"Really? Show me!"

Marc smirked, now somewhat embarrassed.

"Go on, it's okay." I had a foreboding of what was to come.

He glanced toward his dad, who nodded his head. Now with official permission given, Marc began both proudly and awkwardly. "Well, here's some of them: bitch, bastard…" He listed them without voice and Allison did not voice either.[b] Again he looked at his dad who again nodded a go-ahead. Marc resumed, "…stupid, shit, penis, piss, vagina…" He began to giggle and then laugh uncontrollably. Even Laura smirked.

"Do you know those signs, too?" I asked Laura.

"Yeah," she smiled.

"You know what this means?" I asked Laura and Marc. I made the sign for constipation.

"No," they replied in unison. Allison signed their "No" for Debbie and Jim.

"Okay, you guys," I signed to Jim and Debbie, "you explain. You can show its opposite as well." I asked Allison not to voice this time either.

Debbie happily took the lead, beginning with the familiar sign for "shit" that she spatialized to the left. In the middle of her signing space, she made the sign for constipation, now accompanied by contorted facial grimaces; and on the right, she made the sign for "diarrhea" with her tongue hanging out and slouching in her chair. Everybody was in stitches, particularly Laura and Marc. In fact, Marc laughed so hard that he farted. His face turned beet red.

I fingerspelled "f-a-r-t-e-d" to Debbie and pointed to Marc. Without missing a beat, Debbie immediately provided the sign for

---

b. I was about to nonverbally cue Allison not to voice this because voicing it would have ruined the effect. Moreover, I wanted to see if Laura knew these signs. However, Allison discontinued voicing on her own.

fart. Moreover, she also demonstrated some variations or nuances of farting: she used her facial expression and body while changing the speed of her hand movement to depict the slow, painful kind; then she demonstrated the quick kind, then the pleasurable fart and finally what could only be described as the *megafart*.

When Marc finally stopped laughing, he exclaimed, "Mom doesn't let us talk this way."

Jim and Debbie responded with, "You don't have to tell her."

I agreed wholeheartedly, adding that "some secrets are okay!"

Unfortunately, our time was up. It was a great meeting. Clearly, we accomplished much more than laughing or having an ASL tutorial on flatulence. We had begun the task of building important alliances within this recently blended family and of building boundaries between them and the household that included Carol, Marc and Laura's biological mother. The "bricks and mortar" of boundary-making include harmless secrets.

There was more chuckling as we said our goodbyes. Allison and I shared a laugh as well as we began our postsession meeting. We reviewed the communication logistics of the session, specifically the reasons for my cueing her to stop and then resume signing or voicing. As usual, we had been in sync with each other.

The next step with the family was to have a meeting with Jim and his ex-wife, Carol. My goals were several:

1. to set the stage for Carol to more openly permit and encourage the kids to engage with their father and step-mother;
2. to help make it possible for the children to come and go between the two households with greater flexibility (concretely spelled-out visitation schedules may work within the legal system, but their rigidity is often harmful to the children);
3. to acknowledge Jim and Carol as having the primary responsibility for raising their children, thus decreasing Carol's possible defensiveness;
4. to assess whether or not there was an *emotional divorce* between

Jim and Carol. (This is not the case, for example, when a legally divorced couples are not speaking or if they have continuous conflicts. Anger is a very strong bond.)

Jim agreed to a meeting with Carol. He declined my invitation to include an interpreter, saying that "it would be awkward and I can lipread her easily." Two weeks later we met.

Although, as stated in other chapters, where people choose to sit is often not diagnostic, it was noteworthy that Jim and Carol sat on opposite sides of the waiting room; and, once in my office, they chose seats as far away from each other as possible. If my window was open, one of them would undoubtedly have sat on the outside ledge. They were clearly uncomfortable with each other. It was my task to break the ice.

"You have both helped create wonderful children," I began in sim-comm. "They're good and bright kids."

Jim and Carol gave tentative thanks.

I continued. "We're not gathered here today to talk about your marriage or divorce, but to acknowledge your continuing role as co-parents of these wonderful kids of yours." I then proceeded to set up some standard ground rules that I routinely use with divorced couples: namely, that we will stay rigidly focused on their role as coparents with their children and not engage in any renewed versions of the conflicts that had killed their marriage. Both of them nodded their heads and were visibly relieved to hear these safety parameters.

We also set up communication ground rules. We agreed to cue each other before beginning to talk; otherwise, Jim would not be able to track the conversation. We would be sure to talk clearly. I would sim-comm, per Jim's request. And if anything was not clear to Jim, he would immediately get clarification.

The conversation was cordial. Carol had no objection to the kids spending more time with their dad and Debbie, although she had not encouraged them to do so in the past. I asked her why.

Predictably, the tension abruptly escalated. "I think Jim's a very

good father," she began quite tentatively. "But, well, you know—
and I don't mean this to insult you, Jim—but, well, he sometimes
doesn't supervise them enough."

I elicited her concerns in some detail. All of them could be sub-
sumed in the category of safety issues. I decided to take a leap.

"You know, he's not able to hear well."

"Oh really?" she responded with a smile.

"You already knew that, I guess," I smiled back. "But frankly, I
would be somewhat surprised if Jim and Debbie's inability to hear
didn't have something to do with your previous anxiety about your
kids' safety." I purposely used the past tense for her anxiety, although it was also clearly in the present. I needed to be careful not
to negate her earlier statement that she would not object to increased visitation.

"I guess it's part of it," she admitted, now switching back to present tense. But as she elaborated, she emphasized the past. "Particularly when they were younger and we were living together, I was
always scared that Jim couldn't hear them cry. Suppose they hurt
themselves? Suppose they fell down? We had all the visual alarms
and other paraphernalia for deaf people. But, well, I guess I was an
overanxious parent."

"Sometimes being an overanxious parent gets mixed up with feeling comfortable with a deaf spouse," I responded. "But as you say,
you had more fears when they were younger." Rather than give a
sermon, for example, that deaf people often act more safely than do
hearing people—fewer car accidents, etc.—now it was more relevant
to demarcate her fears as belonging to another time.

"That's right," she said.

"Well, since I'm batting a thousand let me go for broke, okay?" I
asked playfully.

"Go for it," she responded, smiling.

"It's also fairly common for one divorced parent to fear that the
kids would be taken away by the other. In your case, I don't mean
anything that would make CNN news, like kidnapping or anything

like that. But perhaps you fear that they might want to only live with Daddy, or that they'll love Daddy more than you, or that they'll sign without talking anymore."

Now Jim lunged forward with "You never wanted them to sign!"

Carol lashed back, "You know—"

"Hold on," I interrupted, realizing that I had obviously hit a nerve. "This is past marital stuff that we agreed to keep off limits. Carol, from this moment on—not yesterday, last month, or last year—what are your current feelings about Marc and Laura learning to sign with their dad and step-mother?"

"I feel fine about it," she assured me.

"I see. But if you hadn't in the past felt as fine about them signing as you do now, what might your reason have been? Because it still might be a factor." Her quick, affirmative response seemed like too neat a package. In this case, I wondered whether the past was, in fact, very much operative in the present.

Now, seeing her ex-husband lean back in his seat and withdraw from combat, she gave my question some thought. "I suppose I didn't want them signing to interfere with them learning to talk."

Jim stiffened and was obviously sitting on strong feelings. "Them signing would have helped their language and speech," he interjected tersely. His expression told me that he had made this statement many times before.

"I agree with you," I assured Jim. "And so does the research. But that was her fear. The Bill of Rights allows people to have irrational fears." We were in danger of straying off the necessary, straight and narrow path of facilitating more present-day engagement between the children and their father.

Looking at Carol, I said, "Well, whether signing would have interfered with their speech or not, the good news is that both of them speak just fine now. They'll have the best of both worlds."

She nodded her head and relaxed. Jim remained still.

"Do you know any signs yourself?" I asked Carol.

Now thrown a little off guard, she hesitantly responded with "I know some."

"Can you sign 'Have fun'?"

She shrugged her shoulders.

"Jim, can you show her?"

Jim dutifully showed her the correct signs, glossed as "You have fun."

"Carol, a great idea would be for you to sign that (without using your voice) to the kids the next time Jim picks them up at the house for a weekend visit. I think they'll get a kick out of it and you'll be giving them a healthy message. It'll also be a sort of peace treaty with Jim. Would you do that?"

"Sure," she smiled. I asked them to practice the sequence a few times.

It was time to stop. I had no grand delusions that everything would be fine after this meeting. But we had hopefully begun a process. Moreover, unlike many divorced couples who have irreconcilable disagreements about child rearing and/or significant emotional disturbance, Jim and Carol seemed genuinely interested and able to cooperate with each other for the sake of their children.

I bid both them goodbye and signed to Carol without voice, "You have fun." She smiled back and, with an "S" hand shape moving up and down, signed "Yes."

***

I met with Jim, Debbie and the three children for about six months. They continued to gain more patience and tolerance of the ambiguity of forming a new, blended family without trying too hard to make everything work out. Family ties do not develop overnight. Another theme was for the parents not to personalize the negative or rejecting reactions of the children, but instead to view their behaviors as part of a normal developmental process—one that can be gratifying and/or frustrating, depending on the day.

I couldn't help but chuckle when I received a card from Debbie and Laura that advertised a fashionable boutique on Newbury Street. Behold the successful therapeutic outcome: increased clothes shopping! Newbury Street should have funded our family therapy visits.

But the outcome of treatment was more than increasing clothing expenditures. Both households had moved beyond the deaf–hearing tug-of-war that had pulled the hearing kids to their hearing mother and away from their deaf father and step-mother. As Laura said on her card, "I like hanging out in Boston because some of the stores are better than in the suburbs. But pizza is better in the burbs."

Rather than having to choose between the Boston or suburban stores, between one parent or the other, or between deaf and hearing loyalties, Laura and Marc could hang out in both worlds, reaping the benefits that each had to offer.

Notes

1. McGoldrick, M., & Carter, B. *Forming a remarried family.*
2. Harvey, M.A. (1989). *Psychotherapy with deaf and hard of hearing persons: A systemic model.* Hillsdale, NJ: Lawrence Erlbaum.
3. Strong, M., & Stone-Charlson, E. (1987). *Simultaneous communication: Are teachers attempting an impossible task?* American Annals of the Deaf, 132(5), 376–382.
4. Harvey, M.A. (1989). *Psychotherapy with deaf and hard of hearing persons: A systemic model.* Hillsdale, NJ: Lawrence Erlbaum.
5. Stansfield, M. (1981). *Psychological issues in mental health interpreting.* R.I.D. Interpreting Journal, 1, 18–32.
6. Taff Watson, M. (1984). Interpreters in mental health settings. In Proceedings of the Fourth Mental Health and Deafness Conference. Toronto, Ontario, Canada: Ontario Institute for Studies in Education.
7. Harvey, M.A. (1989). *Psychotherapy with deaf and hard of hearing persons: A systemic model.* Hillsdale, NJ: Lawrence Erlbaum.
8. Harvey, M.A. (1999). *Odyssey of hearing loss: Tales of triumph.* San Diego, CA: DawnSignPress.

CHAPTER 8

Overcoming Isolation and Despair

"I meet thousands of people surfing the Web!"

Despite Bill's bravado, he didn't sound convincing; in fact, he seemed melancholy. It's not that the Internet *causes* depression, as some newspaper articles would have us believe. It's that it provides one with only a facade of intimacy: communication without eye contact, without potentially awkward goodbyes, and without even the necessity to disclose your identity. An e-mail alias is all that's required. You can divulge your deepest, darkest secrets to endless people you will never meet. Two keyboards passing in cyberspace.

For persons with hearing loss, the Internet also provides a refuge from the loneliness and isolation of being among people whose muffled sounds are impossible to understand. On the computer, every word is crystal clear, limited only by the number of pixels that your video card and monitor can handle. In Internet chat rooms, dialogue happens in orderly sequences, the opposite of the talking-over-each-other stampede that often predominates in groups of hearing people.

However, the Internet is not a replacement for intimacy. Despite Bill's effortless on-line communications with, in his words, "thousands of people across the world," he felt increasingly isolated and lonely. Now in his early 30s and hard-of-hearing since birth, he finally decided to seek psychotherapy one month prior. The dark furrow of his face foreshadowed what he would say next.

"It's pitiful isn't it? Flirting with a computer!"

"What you're saying is that a computer is inadequate to fulfill your social needs. You've been using it not to get information or do spreadsheets, but to flirt or meet people. It's a hell of a tool, but it's *just* a tool."

He thought for a moment, then spoke slowly and deliberately. "It may be just a tool for you, Mike. But for me, it's a lover who's always there for me but who's just out of my reach. I've resigned myself to it."

His metaphor took my breath away. Now on our fourth meeting, he had maintained a taciturn, overintellectualized armor, undoubtedly to prevent me from hurting him, but leaving me feeling only a superficial connection with him. Now, with his defenses temporarily withdrawn, this was my first clear glimpse of his isolation and profound despair. I had an image of a desperate, bereft boy alone on a street corner.

After a pause, I asked him for a point of clarification. "What's the 'it' that you've resigned yourself to?"

"Sitting at home by myself, not having a lover, not going to parties or dances. I was born alone and I'll die alone. It's the human condition and we're all stuck with it. We were thrown out of the Garden of Eden forever! There's nothing unusual about being lonely."

I privately noted his "we are all alone" rationalization to justify his disengagement; it served as more armor to protect him from pain. But there are many who would agree with Bill's assertion. The infamous Adam and Eve story certainly emphasized our having been sentenced to isolation and selfconsciousness. And author Thomas Wolfe wrote that "Loneliness, far from being a rare and curious phenomenon, peculiar to myself and to a few other solitary men, is the central and inevitable fact of human existence." He, too, had resigned himself to solitude: the human condition.[1]

On the other hand, that existential view seems limiting. Psychiatrist Judith Herman, in *Trauma and Recovery,* stated that "while helplessness and isolation are the core experiences of psychological trauma, empowerment and *reconnection* are the core experiences of recovery."[2] In fact, we are *not* born into this world alone; rather, we're biologically connected to our parents. And our psychological growth is inexorably linked to networks of intimate connections. We are social, interdependent creatures who naturally bond with others, so much so that true friendship has been described as "one mind in two bodies."

But this symbiosis is tenuous. Despite our desperate efforts to shed our boundaries and merge with another, we are repeatedly frustrated to find that experiences of "one mind, two bodies" are transitory and remain elusive, just beyond our reach. We are continually catapulted back to the harsh reality of being trapped inside ourselves. Although we are social creatures, we nevertheless are alone.

This paradox is the essence of the human condition, said psychoanalyst Eric Erikson. He explained that our psychological development hinges on how we manage what he called "a dynamic balance of opposites [of] two seemingly contrary dispositions." Our fundamental psychological task, beginning most prominently in young adulthood, is to balance the "contrary dispositions" of being *social* versus *alone;* or, in their extremes, merger versus detachment. If we are successful, we are then able to achieve intimacies outside of our immediate families, and simultaneously achieve a more expansive sense of ourselves.

However, for many people with hearing losses, this essential balance becomes lopsided toward detachment. Leaving the structure of school and home may not lead to participating in expanding social networks and developing an expanded self; rather it may lead to isolation, despair, and "loss of self." Bill recounted a common scenario: "Going to parties is sheer hell for me. Once in a while I make myself go, or my friends will say what a great party it'll be. But I always get real down about it. And once I finally get there, it sucks!"

Bill was shaking his head. He was apparently reliving or recalling a painful ordeal.

"I remember one time talking with some people who've known me for several years and knew I was hard-of-hearing. But they kept forgetting. I don't know why. I kept reminding them. I don't hide my hearing aids behind my hair like some people do. But they think I do great and that I function fine. My speech is good, so what's the big deal! But it's much more subtle than that."

"Please go on," I prompted him. He was letting me inside his hellish world.

"They don't get it!" he yelled. "When people are talking, it isn't just the words that I'm trying to understand. I'm trying to figure out peoples' facial expressions, body language, the subtle stuff that they mutter under their breaths and other innuendoes. And jokes, forget it! I may hear the beginning of a joke, the slow part. But the punch line is usually fast and muffled. There's no way I can get it. And it stilts the conversation if I ask them to repeat the punch line. So I laugh, too, just to be polite.

"Once when I finally told someone that I'm hard-of-hearing and can't get everything in noisy groups. That asshole had the bloody nerve to say to me that 'you know, I'm also hard-of-hearing at parties; with a bunch of noise and commotion, who isn't?'"

"What does he know?" Bill screamed to the wall as if "that asshole" were in my office. "It takes every last ounce of my concentration," Bill continued as he composed himself. "If someone says something—let's say 'best'—it's hard for me understand the letter S. So I think he said 'bet.' It sounds logical. But a few minutes later, something in our conversation—I'm not sure what—doesn't quite make sense. I obviously missed something, but I don't know what and I don't know when. So I can't ask the person about it. Then I feel inadequate and try harder to watch the words. But it's a catch-22: The more I watch for the words, the more I miss other stuff that people communicate. And here again, I'm lost. I constantly feel left out."

"Let me see if I get this," I said. "You start off feeling left out, so you focus on the words. You get some of the words, but then you end up feeling even more left out than before because you miss the subtle but equally important levels of communication?"

"You got it!" he replied.

"And then what happens?"

"As the night wears on, I get more and more stressed. My stress takes away whatever is left of my concentration. So the more stressed I feel, the more I can't hear. I sort of go on automatic pilot, keeping my end of the conversation—smiling when they smile, nodding my head every once in a while. Then I say to myself, 'How did I get myself in this mess anyway?' I wish I could disappear, escape, or that someone would beam me up someplace. To be honest with you, Mike, it's an utterly overwhelming and terrifying experience."

I nodded my head. "In those situations, do you typically imagine a place where you would like to be beamed up to?" (We were both Star Trek fans.)

"Where I can relax."

"And where's that?" I asked.

"Home in front of my computer with a bottle of bourbon. At least then I don't have to feel so shitty about myself."

Like some hard-of-hearing persons who retreat from the world, Bill befriended not only his computer but alcohol as well. A fifth of Jack Daniels, like his e-mail acquaintances, would understand his deepest wishes and fears. The bourbon would also sufficiently anesthetize Bill so he wouldn't have to suffer his loneliness so deeply. But his respite was only temporary. As he came to realize that e-mail partners (and alcohol) were only pseudointimate relationships, he was confronted with the reality that the balance of his social-alone needs swayed dangerously toward detachment and isolation. He was in a lot of pain.

"In what way do you feel shitty?" I asked.

"People talking too fast makes me feel inferior," Bill stated.

An instant, knee-jerk reflex came out of my mouth. "No one has the power to make you feel anything." I went on to quote Eleanor Roosevelt's saying, "No one can make you feel inferior without your consent."[3] I wanted to emphasize what he *could* control, that he wasn't completely helpless with respect to his thoughts and feelings. Perhaps it was my desperate attempt to offer him a quick cure.

"That's a bunch of crap, Doc," Bill fired back. "It's easy for you to say," he continued. "How would you feel if you stood in the middle of a crowd, everyone was having an animated discussion—arguing, sharing stories, laughing at jokes, making new friends—and you couldn't understand a goddamn thing they said! You mean to tell me you wouldn't feel just a wee bit inferior? Give me a break." His voice shifted to convey a volatile mixture of irritation and hurt.

Bill was right. On the one hand, it certainly made sense that any person would feel "just a wee bit inferior" in such conversationally inaccessible and isolating environments for the reasons he had listed. It's not that his formulation—that a situation *causes* one to feel inferior—was wrong; it was *incomplete*. I recall a quotation by Henry Brooks Adams. "No man likes to have his intelligence or good faith questioned, especially if he already has doubts about it himself."[4]

What were Bill's prior doubts about himself? And how did these doubts set the stage for him to feel inferior in party environments? My first step was to lay the groundwork for exploring some answers to these complicated questions. Then we would forge tools that would help undo the damage done to Bill by years of emotional isolation.

"You know," I began, "it's as if that party situation both contributes to your self-doubt and also reactivates earlier memories of self-doubt and selfdepreciation. If your cup is already half-full with inferiority, then it won't take too much additional stress to cause it to overflow."

I borrowed that metaphor from the allergy/asthma literature. If you're already suffering from mild asthma because of allergies and then come in contact with an additional allergen (e.g., a cat), you might then have a full-blown asthma attack. But the cat would not

be the sole cause of the attack. Rather, the addition of the cat allergen to your already almost full "asthma cup" would cause it to overflow. Stated differently, if you were protected from all the other
environmental allergens and therefore had an "empty cup" while in
contact with the cat, you would suffer little or no asthma.

Bill thought for a moment and his countenance softened. He was
a dual computer and English major in college and also enjoyed playing with words. He often called me a frustrated Bob Newhart, in
reference to Newhart's television role as a psychologist who also rev-
eled in using analogies and metaphors. In a more playful manner he
asked "Is that sort of like saying 'your plate is half-full and you can't
put too much more on it?'"

I laughed and responded, "You can use plates, if you want; but
with food on them, not water."

Bill, obviously enjoying the poetic distraction from his displeas-
ure with me, then offered a third metaphor. "Like when I'm operating too many programs with insufficient RAM?"

"Go on," I smiled.

"You know, let's say you have only 64 megabytes of available
RAM. If you're running software that requires, let's say, 50
megabytes of memory and then boot up a program that requires an
additional 20 megabytes, then the last program will crash. But if you
close all the other programs, it'll run just fine."

"No experience exists in isolation," I said thinking out loud.
"Each of our thoughts, feelings, behaviors and perceptions are *hy-
perlinked* to each other so that when any one 'Web site' is accessed,
several others are simultaneously activated. Our sense of self and the
world are linked or wired to previous scenes in our lives. There are
always more people in the room than we immediately see. I just
thought of another metaphor! Maybe—"

"I get the point, Doc," Bill interrupted. He called me "Doc"
when I became too pedantic.

"I was just getting warmed up," I complained. "You're going to
make me feel bad."

"I can't make you feel anything," he answered.

We both laughed. But we knew we had returned to an uneasy point of contention.

"Tell me if this thinking pattern sounds familiar," I continued. "'I don't understand the muffled sounds around me at parties not only because of my defective ears, but also because of my defective intelligence, defective character, defective personality, defective self, defective soul—in short, because I'm a worthless piece of scum who has no business taking up space on planet Earth with nondefective homo sapiens.'"

Bill's back abruptly stiffened. "What I think," he responded with renewed irritation "is that I can't understand people because I'm hard-of-hearing. It's—"

"It's bullshit, you—"

"You don't think I'm hard-of-hearing?" Bill interrupted.

"I know you're hard-of-hearing. That's an undisputed fact. But if you only thought to yourself at parties, 'I'm hard-of-hearing, therefore I sometimes can't understand conversation,' you wouldn't feel inferior, like a worthless piece of scum." My voice was getting louder.

"It's damn frustrating not to be able to function well in groups." By this time, he was also raising his voice. No more poetic distraction; we were having a good fight.

"No shit," I yelled back. "Of course, it's frustrating. But it'll help to be very specific about how much you're able to hear: what expectations you have of yourself."

"What do you mean?"

In a softer voice, I responded to his sincere question. "With a moderate hearing loss, exactly how much do you expect to understand? One hundred percent? Eighty? Fifty? Twenty?"

"How do I know?" Bill responded with more annoyance.

"How the hell do *I* know?" I echoed, this time with attempted playful compassion.

"I don't understand your question," he said, still obviously angry.

"It's a simple question really, although it sounds confusing. You may not realize it, but you have, at some level, an expectation that you'll understand a certain percentage of other peoples' speech. If you expect, for example, to understand *all* conversation, you're bound to fall short and feel frustrated. On the other hand, if you expect to understand *no* conversation—zero percent—then you're bound to greatly surpass your objective and will feel elated. Your percentage should be somewhere in between."

"Well, I don't think about choosing a percentage when I go to parties," Bill said, persisting in his annoyance.

"I bet you do," I also persisted, "but probably not consciously."

Adjustment to hearing loss largely depends on how much access to information you expect to have; on trying to maximize your accessibility to information while tolerating the inevitable reduced accessibility. Suppose, for example, full access to information is impossible in a given situation. There are at least three solutions: (a) increase your efforts at all costs, (b) avoid the situation, or (c) try your best and accept partial success. The first option results in frustration, the second in isolation. Researchers Kyle and Wood suggest the third option. "The degree to which an individual can tolerate reduced and varying access to information [in one's environment] will determine the degree of adjustment."[5]

My task with Bill was to help him determine what level of reduced information flow he was willing to tolerate. A simple homework task: I asked him to attend a group function for a duration of at least four hours and to monitor his level of self-confidence under four consecutive one-hour conditions. Condition 1 would be for him to have a conscious expectation of understanding 100% of conversation; condition 2 was with a reduced expectation of only understanding 75% of conversation; and conditions 3 and 4 were 50 and 25% expectations, respectively. I further asked him to estimate how much conversation he actually understood under each condition.

Predictably, Bill experienced marked frustration in the 100 and 75% conditions. In each case, he felt he understood only about 40%

and his self-confidence plummeted; in his words, "I felt really shitty about myself." He felt much more confident, however, in the 50 and 25% conditions. Interestingly, in both of these conditions, he estimated being able to understand 60% of conversation! *Bill understood more when he was not trying so hard!*

The ripple effects of Bill reducing his expectations of informational accessibility were: (1) it caused his frustration and stress to decrease, (2) it caused his self confidence to increase, and (3) it caused his perception of how much he understood to *increase.*

"So I should settle and expect less?" Bill asked somewhat sarcastically.

"You should hope and work for nirvana but expect to end up somewhere on Earth, between heaven and hell," I responded.

I have observed that an all-or-nothing, thinking pattern is common with persons who have disability: namely, the supposition that if their disability cannot be completely mastered, it will hinder not *some but all* aspects of their competency. In this framework, given that the handicapping effects of a disability are typically impossible to completely eliminate, humiliation and failure are practically guaranteed. This disempowered stance is opposite to the intent of the popular Deaf-affirmative slogan, "The only thing Deaf people can't do is hear."

Bill attached several negative attributes to his hearing loss that went beyond its inevitable audiological ramifications. Instead, his negativity defined his view of himself as totally defective and inferior. By "filling his cup" with these self-condemnations, he put himself at risk for feeling inferior at group gatherings. It was his pattern of thinking that *caused* him to feel inferior; "people talking too fast" was not the culprit. Losing self-confidence in conversationally inaccessible situations is a version of blaming the victim, only here, the victim blames him/herself.

It was time to more directly address Bill's self-condemnation. We would then substitute more realistic and helpful ways of thinking. "Part of the solution does have to do with you consciously specifying exactly how much information you expect to understand in any given environment—somewhere between zero and one hundred percent—and feeling satisfied with that: 'settling,' as you put it. But it's much easier said than done. It's not that simple."

"Nothing seems simple anymore," Bill complained, now seeming less angry and irritated but more overwhelmed.

"Important things tend not to be simple," I said trying to comfort him. "I wish I knew why, but life's profound lessons always seem complicated. And one very important, nonsimple task is to figure out what's in your cup or that you're using up too much RAM. Because it's this stuff that gets activated when you're conversationally lost; and it's this stuff that *makes* you feel inferior."

Silence permeated the room. I felt that we were just beginning to enter a deeper level of Bill's world that had been so far oversimplified by our metaphors of asthma cups and RAM.

"What are you thinking?" I finally asked.

"I remember my mom and dad convincing me to go to the Panthorama, my ninth-grade dance. It was a Friday night and the high school gym was decorated with crepe paper, balloons, tinsel, and ribbon, all with orange and green, the school colors. A bunch of the "in" crowd was there: Laurie, Marji, Betty, Rhonda, and even Shelly, who was the head cheerleader and the queen of the clique. Shelly was absolutely gorgeous! And the band's music was blasting away through their new Fender amps."

He paused. "I didn't want to go but my parents said I would have a good time. They even bribed me with twenty bucks! But you know the end of the story," Bill sighed as he looked down toward the floor."

"Dark, noisy, crowded place, huh?"

"You got it," Bill said.

"And what did that experience put in your cup?" I asked.

"Well, I was never a good dancer, so I ended up standing by the potato chip and Kool-Aid table." Bill then hesitated for a second and took a deep breath, apparently to prepare himself for what would be a painful disclosure. "I noticed Shelly coming toward me and my heart practically jumped out of my chest. She came to the table to get a drink, noticed me and said something. But I couldn't understand her. She repeated it. I still couldn't understand her. So she shook her head in disgust and walked away."

Shaking his head, he muttered, "I felt like a pariah."

A not-so-unusual but excruciatingly painful experience. But for Bill, it felt unique only to him; he judged that it was his hearing loss that repelled and disgusted Shelly. After all, it was his hearing loss that had prevented him from understanding her speech amidst the Fender amps. Indeed, his assumption may or may not have been correct; maybe Shelly reacted negatively to having to repeat herself. But Bill's assumption didn't stop there. He also judged that it was his body, mind, and soul that were repulsive to Shelly; why else would she have walked away? Moreover, he then concluded that he must be repulsive, a pariah. At that time, barely 14 years old, he didn't have the cognitive tools to view himself any other way.

I asked him if he had other associations or memories that also evoked a sense of himself as repulsive. He needed no prompting; there were already too many additional stories crowded in his consciousness. These included school plays in "echo-chamber auditoriums," Thanksgiving dinners with hoards of relatives, and Christmas gatherings when family and friends would sit around the tree with loud caroling filling the room—loud, crowded environments.

"With reference to these situations—the party, plays, Thanksgiving, Christmas, et cetera—what did you think to yourself about yourself?" I asked.

"I didn't think anything except 'let me outta here.'"

"But you also thought something about you. You mentioned pariah." It would be important to elicit Bill's negative self-talk, since present-day acoustically inaccessible environments triggered it to erupt in full force.

"I felt like there was something wrong with me—that I was defective, stupid, inferior."

"You thought that, not felt it," came my seemingly picky re-minder. I wanted to set the stage for us to focus on his thinking pat-terns as the primary causal agents for his feelings. The phrase "something is wrong with me" is a *thought* that then causes you to *feel* depressed.

"Now for the crucial question: If those earlier situations—and undoubtedly many others like them—had not happened, would crowds of hearing people 'make' you feel inferior in the present?"

"Probably not," he conceded, after giving it some thought. "But these experiences *did* happen. So I'm stuck, given that I can't rewrite history."

"You can't rewrite your history, but you can rewrite what you have allowed your history to teach you about yourself and your world, what assumptions you make."

"What do you mean?" he asked.

"Certain things inevitably happen. If I'm sick, I'll be tired. If it's dark, I won't be able to see. If it's too light, I'll squint. But ac-knowledging my limitations doesn't have to mean thinking that there's something wrong with me, that I'm defective, stupid, or in-ferior. It does mean, however, that I have to grieve the loss of fanta-sized omnipotence. Only superman can jump tall buildings with a single bound, not human beings. As humans, we have to hold on to our self-esteem when we can't do certain things. It's bad enough being frustrated without giving away our competence."

I observed myself getting on my Cognitive Behavioral Therapy soapbox, preparing to pontificate that thoughts cause feelings that then may cause certain behaviors. Bill's thoughts included the no-tions that his failure to understand a certain percentage and other facets of conversation meant that he was inferior, "pathetic," and "like a pariah"; and that other people physically or symbolically walking away from him—the "Shellys" of the world—meant that he deserved that sentence. It would be vital to emphasize that Bill *had a choice* of whether to continue thinking this way. Then he would be more able to negotiate the demands and reap the psychological benefits of being alone and connecting with others.

There are important benefits from deepening our solitary and social experiences, *provided that they are proportionally balanced over time.*[a] Being alone invites us to become immersed in uninterrupted streams of consciousness and to think out loud without anyone's censure. We then encounter deeper levels of our being; in a sense, we become our own best friend. We master a critical developmental task: to be alone without feeling lonely.

Our success at this task, however, necessarily depends on mastering another critical task: namely, to be social without necessarily giving away our identity. Being social invites us to try on "different hats," to be in Rome and do as the Romans do; to allow another to lead us beyond our own self-circumscribed world. Being social invites opportunities for us to learn empathy as we try to stand in another's shoes; and it enables us to know ourselves through other people, what they may perceive in us that we do not.

The capacities to be alone and social are interdependent. We often don't see that how we relate to another inevitably follows from how we relate to ourselves, that our outer relationships are an extension of our inner life. Similarly, how we relate to ourselves inevitably follows from how we have related to other key people in our lives. As Bill was soon to discover, these others have the capacity to become psychologically present within us when we are alone.

Another key benefit of balancing these contrary opposites is that we learn how to maintain an even sense of self-competence despite any stressors. Even if others are kicking me—assaulting my self-esteem—I can nevertheless protect and comfort myself. I call it being "psychologically warm blooded": despite a warm or cold environ-

---

a. There does not have to be a daily a priori defined ratio of alone and social time. On the contrary, many people profitably go through periods of time engaged in heightened socialization; others in heightened solitude. Rather, per a major tenet of Erikson's framework, there needs to be a *cumulative* balance of these contrary dispositions over the course of one's life.

ment, the "temperature" of our own self-esteem remains constant.

"Don't let them take your self-esteem. Hold on to it!" I said to Bill.

"Easier said than done. Just how do I hold on to my self-esteem in impossible-to-function-in, hearing environments?"

"You need to look at what's already in your cup and put something or someone else in it. You can't get rid of the negative, distressing voices. But I would suggest the following: Imagine someone in your past, present, or who you may meet in the future. It could be a fictional character, someone on TV, in a book, or in the movies—anyone who could with credibility soothe you—who, if he or she were there during the Panthorama with Shelly, at Thanksgiving, Christmas, and at other parties, would comfort you, someone who would enable you to hold on to who you are, who would prevent you from giving your self-esteem away."

He seemed intrigued and immersed himself in thought for several moments. "Mrs. Thomas was my sixth-grade teacher. Although I wasn't the best student in her class, I think she liked me. She would ask how I'm doing. And I can still hear her saying, 'Good job, Bill. I'm really proud of you.'"

He said it one more time, this time nodding his head slightly with the beginnings of a child-like smile. "'Good job, Bill. I'm really proud of you.'"

"Can you see her in your mind's eye?" I asked.

"Yeah, I can see her smile, her always neat gray hair and she usually wore a bright-colored kerchief around her neck. She seemed real tall, at least to me as a kid."

"We all need a Mrs. Thomas," I said softly.

He nodded, this time more definitively.

"You may not be able to 'beam' yourself away from parties but you can, at least in your head, beam Mrs. Thomas to you. You can have private discussions with her."

It was time to do one of my favorite guided imageries, one that I personally use in times of stress when I need to talk to someone who is not physically present. After some standard preparation—making sure he was comfortable, doing deep breathing and relaxation exercises—we were ready to begin.

"Bill, after I finish speaking, I'd like you to close your eyes and find Mrs. Thomas. Do a file search. Perhaps you'll see her, hear her voice, smell her fragrance, or feel her pat you on the back. And when you open your eyes, I'd like you to tell Mrs. Thomas what gifts she had given to you, gifts that no one can ever take away, gifts that you can also summon or 'beam up' in times of need."

Bill closed his eyes, lay back in his seat and took a deep breath. He had a look of contentment that I hadn't seen before. He was in a special, loving, nurturing place, one known only to him. We all have our own special places that we can privately go to in times of need, when we want to be comforted and told that everything is okay.

I thought of my daughter's once favorite television show, Pippi Longstocking. It was about a young red-headed girl whose father had left many years ago to go off to sea. In times of need, Pippi would stand by the ocean talking to "The Captain." He would talk to Pippi through the waves; and no matter how badly she had been feeling, she would end up knowing that she was okay, that she was a good and lovable person.

Bill opened his eyes. I motioned to him to place Mrs. Thomas—his version of The Captain—in the chair across from him and to talk to her.

At first, he squirmed in his seat, obviously thinking this was either silly or perhaps deeply personal. But after only a little encouragement, he began:

> "Mrs. Thomas, I know I have never told you this. I guess as a kid, I was too shy and didn't know the right words. Maybe I thought it would be sissyish and the other kids would overhear and laugh at me."

He paused, obviously struggling to find the right words.

"The other kids aren't here; and I won't tell them," I interjected.

Looking straight at the chair, he then said:

> I want to thank you for believing in me, for noticing me, for showing me that I deserved your attention and that my broken ears didn't mean I was a broken person. I never thanked you for that. You have no idea how important what you did was.

"Tell her," I said softly.

"I can still hear you saying to me, 'You can rise above it, you can rise above it.' You would put your hand on my shoulder; and it made me feel that I was okay." Bill began to sob.

I was moved by how deeply Mrs. Thomas had touched Bill and how he was allowing her to continue touching him, even though she perhaps had long since physically passed away. We also both smiled in reference to his purposeful emphasis of *"made me feel."*

"I agree," I said, now with tears in my eyes. "You beaming up Mrs. Thomas does, in fact, *cause* you to hold on to your self-esteem no matter where you are. And it's a lot better for your liver than Jack Daniels."

Bill nodded his head emphatically. "And you don't even get a hangover!"

We both laughed and exchanged a warm glance. "You can bring her to parties with you, you know. You can bring her to future Thanksgivings, Christmas gatherings—anywhere you want. And if you bring her to the movies or theater, you don't even need to buy an extra ticket."

"I know," he smiled. "I just wish I had known that before. But at least I know it now."

"I wonder what will happen when Shelly and Mrs. Thomas meet?" I half-seriously asked, changing the subject.

"Yeah, right," he said dismissively.

"No, I'm serious. You already, perhaps unconsciously, bring Shelly with you in your head to parties and to other impossible-to-function-in group gatherings. That's partially why you have felt so crappy about yourself. When you also bring Mrs. Thomas, they will undoubtedly meet. Perhaps you should formally introduce them to each other beforehand." We exchanged a mischievous smile.

"Okay, Doc, and just how are we to arrange this meeting?"

I had become "Doc" again, this time not due to my pedantics but undoubtedly because of the science fiction, "Back to the Future" nature of my suggestion. "You don't have to build a time machine. You can arrange them to meet any night when you're asleep."

"This isn't one of your analogies, is it?" he groaned.

"No, not this time," I laughed. "Arrange for Shelly and Mrs. Thomas to meet in your dreams. And watch what happens."

I was quite serious. There is an Indian tribe in New Guinea, the Senoi Indians, who have made "creative dreaming" a sacred part of their daily rituals. Every morning, they sit in a circle and recount their dreams from the previous night; and then plan for what they will dream the following night.[6] I asked Bill to fall asleep thinking about Shelly and Mrs. Thomas having a conversation.

Several weeks later, Bill recounted the following dream:

"I was at my company's Christmas party, sort of standing around feeling stupid. And this beautiful goddess-like woman with long, flowing hair accidentally bumped into me and spilled my bourbon. She said 'I'm sorry' or something but I couldn't get all of it. It was Shelly! She began to make fun of me, said something to her friends and walked away.

"Then I went to the bar for another drink. But the bartender was Mrs. Thomas! She said, 'Bill you don't need any more bourbon. But here's some orange juice.' Orange juice! After what Shelly did to me?

"I expected her to say 'rise above it' but this time, she located Shelly across the room and yelled to her 'Come back here you bitch!' (It shocked me to see sweet old Mrs. Thomas get so angry). Her voice was crystal clear to me but, ironically, now it was Shelly who couldn't hear her above the noise. She yelled again; but Shelly still couldn't hear her. So Mrs. Thomas magically appeared in front of her.

"'How dare you treat Bill that way,' she scolded Shelly. 'He deserves much more than that. He's a sensitive, bright, funny, handsome young man. And whatever problem you have with people who have disabilities, rise above it!'

"Then they began talking about something that, even in my dream, I couldn't understand over the music. But after their talk, Shelly came over and asked me to dance. No conversation; just to dance. Then she smiled and I noticed that some of her teeth were crooked. But she was still beautiful, even with crooked teeth.

"As we danced, she suddenly split into two halves: half remained as Shelly and the other half became Mrs. Thomas. The three of us held hands and twirled round and round. But then, I also split into two halves: and half of me remained on the dance floor and my other half was somewhere near the ceiling looking down at us. I was floating above the whole party, making observations, taking it all in. And then I woke up."

***

Our remaining sessions focused on helping Bill develop the skills to "rise above it" and to consciously converse not only with Shelly but with Mrs. Thomas in potentially ego-deflating situations. As his dream suggested, we cannot get rid of our negative self-talk; "Shelly-ectomies" are impossible. But we can supplement such negativity with positive self-talk and have a productive dialogue in our head.

Bill's balance of social and alone time gradually shifted away from isolation. He attended some parties, although they continued to be largely frustrating for him; his hearing loss precluded his under-standing much of the social chatter. But he expected that. And with the help of a comforting and affirmative inner dialogue, he was able, for the most part, to hang on to his self-esteem. Thus, he often man-aged to find an oasis where he could truly enjoy himself.

Each of us has our own version of a Mrs. Thomas in our soul if we would only look long enough. Our Mrs. Thomas looks over us, helps us in times of need and makes sure that we are *never really alone.* All we have to do is find her.

Notes

1. Wolfe, T. (cited in 1994). The Speaker's Electronic Reference Collection, A Apex Software.
2. Herman, J. (1992). *Trauma and recovery.* New York: Basic Books.
3. Roosevelt, E. (1936). *The wit and wisdom of Eleanor Roosevelt.* New York: Alec Ayres.
4. Adams, H.B. from website http://www.quotegallery.com/asp/allaquotes. asp?author=Henry+Brooks+Adams.
5. Kyle, J. G., Jones, L. G., & Wood, P. C. (1985). Adjustment to acquired hearing loss: A working model. *In* H. Orlans (Ed.), *Adjustment to adult hearing loss.* San Diego, CA: College-Hill Press.
6. Garfield, P. L. (1995). *Creative dreaming.* New York: Fireside.

CHAPTER 9

Leaving Home

I hadn't heard from Tom since Nancy's death six years before (see Chapter 4, An Interrupted Story). He called me one morning at exactly 10:50, remembering that there would be a greater chance of getting me at ten-of-the-hour. Sure enough, I was between appointments. Perhaps to jog my memory of who he was, he asked me whether "anyone else had ever thrown coffee in your office?" I replied truthfully that that honor belonged to him alone and gave Tom a fond hello. Now on a more somber note, he told me that it would have been his 24th wedding anniversary with Nancy that day.

Tom then summarized some important recent events in his life. He had been in individual psychotherapy for several years and had come to understand how, in his words, "a bunch of childhood stuff was, in fact, alive and well in the present"—influences that, like many of us, he had mistakenly assumed were forever locked up in his distant past. He had taken a hard look at his depression, workaholism, and existential and spiritual goals. He joined Amnesty International as a conscious way of "giving back to humanity and making my life sacred." Nancy had joined that organization just one month before she died. He then added, with a hint of awkwardness, that he had been living with a woman for the past year.

As my 10-minute window between appointments was about to end, he got to the point of his phone call. He was concerned about his daughter, Alice. Now in her mid-20s, she had graduated from a collaborative high school program for deaf students with barely a C average and a seventh-grade reading level. As the audiologist correctly predicted many years before, she had learning disabilities, secondary to meningitis, specifically mild attentional deficits and dyslexia. Her hearing had deteriorated from a moderate hearing loss and was now in the "almost profound" range. Currently, she was living with Tom and his partner, had withdrawn socially and was not working; she remained "glued to the couch all day and all night." He wanted me to see Alice for individual therapy.

I responded that it would be my pleasure, provided that Alice herself wanted to meet with me. It often, although not always, does little or no good to see clients who are coerced into your office. We made a tentative appointment for the following week.

Alice showed up in my waiting room 15 minutes late "because of traffic." She gave me a limp handshake in an apologetic or passive manner, I couldn't tell which. Her dress was rumpled although clean. She displayed a listless affect with no sign of a smile or animation. Once in my office, she slumped in the middle of the couch as far down as her body would take her, gluing herself to the fixture like her father had described her doing at home. With stark blankness, she waited for me to begin.

Typically my first question with persons who have a significant or profound hearing loss has to do with our communication. Remembering that she had been exposed to sign language in high school, I listed some options: I could talk and sign at the same time, sign without voice or talk without signing. Using simultaneous communication—voice and sign—she responded that "sim-comm is fine." Her signing was clear and her voice barely intelligible.

"I remember your mother very well," I began in sim-comm. "It was an awful tragedy."

"Thanks," Alice responded, now making eye contact with me for the first time. "I sort of remember your phone call when I told you she died. I still miss her a lot."

"I bet you do. She was a very special person." Alice and I obviously connected around her mother. I, too, had very fond memories of Nancy; and I, too, felt betrayed by her death. "What do you miss about her the most?" I asked.

"She used to help me a lot with homework," Alice said with the beginnings of tears in her eyes.

"She was a good mother." I felt Alice's sadness. She would later tell me that it was her mother who comforted her when she came home from school in tears because the hearing kids ignored or mocked her. Her mother attended every IEP meeting, whereas her father was typically "at work." She persistently advocated for the school program to provide extra tutorial services and extra speech therapy as well as for the school to guarantee including sign language interpreters for all of her mainstream classes.

In contrast, Tom, her father, had always been a distant, amorphous figure, whose presence was laced with an approach-avoidance awkwardness that, to this day, Alice didn't understand. "I don't know why," she said, "but he was never involved much."

I found myself wondering whether Tom had told her about the times in his childhood that he had described to me. The time when he spent "an eternity" waiting for his mother to comfort him after his roller skating accident as a seven-year-old kid and about his own emotionally distant father whose fledgling attempts to provide comfort were only to tell him not to cry (see Chapter 4, An Interrupted Story).

Similarly, Alice, throughout her childhood, repeatedly approached her dad, almost begging him to pay more attention to her—in her words, "more than just taking me out for ice cream." But her efforts were often to no avail. And it was again her mom who would nurse her wounds of rejection, this time, however, not from insensitive hearing peers but from her dad. Her mother was the knight, the consoler, the protector, the one who continually gave Alice the strength to withstand repeated social and familial rejections. She would give Alice the strength to get back on her feet and "enter the ring again."

Without any apparent shame, Alice remembered, "When I heard that my mom got killed in a car accident, I wished that it could have been my dad." A poignant pause. Interestingly, for her confession, Alice had switched communication modality to a more American Sign Language syntax and turned off her voice. Perhaps she felt more comfortable with me and/or ASL was a more primary and preferred language for her than was English. I followed suit, also signing ASL with voice-off. I would ask her later about her language preference.

"It must have been very hard," I affirmed in ASL. It's quite normal, albeit "politically incorrect," to wish that one parent would die before the other. I admired her courage to openly admit it.

We then discussed whether she would like to set up some psychotherapy meetings with me and what she would like to work on. Alice replied affirmatively and that she would like to "talk about what to do with my life." Happily, it was a goal that she and her father shared. He would fund her therapy beyond what third-party insurance payments would cover.

"Can you tell me more specifically what 'getting on with your life' would look like? What would you be doing?" I asked.

"I don't know," she responded.

"Any ideas?"

"Maybe get a job somewhere." She told me that she had worked at a pizza parlor for several months but quit for reasons that were not clear at present.

"That's a good beginning," I responded. "I'd be happy to meet with you and we can discuss the next steps in your life." She nodded her head. We scheduled a series of weekly appointments.

As Alice left, I found myself ruminating on my interrupted work with her parents. What would have been different for Alice if her mother hadn't died? How did Tom's previous emotional disengagement from the family affect Alice? What factors lead her to her present predicament of being "glued to the couch" without direction or confidence? There had to be a reason. But then I laughed at my growing irritation with these unanswered questions, recalling an account of the Dalai Lama's critique of Western psychiatry:

> In some instances, the basic premises and parameters set up by Western science can limit your ability to deal with certain realities. For instance, you have the constraints of the idea that... everything can and must be explained and accounted for. But when you encounter phenomena that you cannot account for, then there's a kind of a tension created, its almost a feeling of agony.[1]

Maybe wisdom is the art of continuing to ask questions but without expecting answers.

Alice showed up late for her next appointment, this time because of "oversleeping." As her story unfolded, it became clear that she was quite ambivalent about becoming independent. On the one hand, she expected her dad or his partner to cook all her meals (although once in a while she would get her own cereal and milk for breakfast) and she seldom volunteered to clean up the dishes. She didn't wash her clothes, or make her bed, or clean up her messes. And until a couple of weeks ago when her dad bought her a car, she depended on him for transportation. She indicated with a hint of shame that "I don't know how to do a lot of stuff."

On the other hand, she admonished her dad for "controlling me too much and telling me what to do all the time." She also charged him with "never leaving me alone." After receiving any major advice from him—i.e., how to write a resume, how to dress for a job interview, where to go shopping for bargains, why she needed to take the antibiotics for the full 10 days—she would check with her girlfriend as to whether her dad's advice was sound. Alice ended her long list of grievances by reporting, with obvious consternation, that he "even picked my car for me. It wasn't the one I wanted; it was the wrong color!"

Frankly, on hearing her complaints, my first goal was to be supportive and not to laugh. After all, Tom had paid a fair amount of money for a good used car; had done all the negotiations with the seller; and, against Alice's vehement protests, Tom had insisted that they get the car checked out by a certified mechanic before purchasing it. (Her girlfriend had rendered her definitive judgement that the car inspection was unnecessary). But I reminded myself that much of her resentment of Tom was undoubtedly reflective of her previous sense of abandonment by him and their current awkwardness with each other. Moreover, she still depended on her dad but resented it terribly: so-called *hostile dependence.* Alice had a double-whammy: she had to come to terms with not only the sudden departure of her mother but with the sudden and perhaps ambiguous emergence of her father.

One of Tom's goals in buying Alice a car was to enable her to expand her job search beyond walking or biking distance from home. He had also scheduled a meeting for Alice with the state vocational rehabilitation agency and an independent living center for Deaf clients, so that she would learn "life skills," such as keeping a check book, budgeting, and utilizing community services. In addition, Tom was concerned about her social withdrawal as a result of always being glued to the couch.

"Although you really wanted a green car instead of the gray one that he bought you," I began, "what plans do you have for it?"

"I don't know," came her response.

"Any ideas?" I persisted.

"Well, you know, I'll drive around."

"Any ideas where?"

"Well, there's a bar in Brighton that a lot of deaf people go to every Thursday night. Maybe I'll go there."

"And what do you hope will happen if you go there?"

"Maybe I'll see some old friends of mine. A lot of them graduated high school with me and I haven't seen them in a long time."

"That's a great idea!" I replied, with deliberate enthusiasm. My hope was that Alice getting out of the house would not only expand her social life beyond one friend but that she would meet other peers who were getting on with their lives. Perhaps they would motivate her to earn more money via some kind of employment or even take classes somewhere. I wished her good luck.

Alice came in for her next week's appointment quite jubilant and on time. She did in fact visit the bar and meet some old friends. But she had an unexpected adventure.

"When I went to find my car, it wasn't there!"

"Where was it?"

"Well, it got towed."

"I see. And why did it get towed?"

"Well, I guess I parked it in a tow zone."

This time I openly laughed, and told her of a similar experience of my own. I couldn't help but frame her unexpected adventure as one of a long list of educational opportunities that would be presented to her. "It sounds like you got an added benefit of learning one important lesson about life: where to park. No parking in tow zones."

"Yeah, I know that now," she admitted. "My friends helped me find it. But I had to pay the towing company money to give my car back to me," she complained with outrage.

Two steps forward, one backward. Although Alice was chronologically 24 years old, it was like talking to an adolescent. She had a naivete about the world that was obvious to other people but to which she was oblivious. However, I complimented her on taking the initiative to unglue herself from the couch and for locating her car. That was progress. She thanked me for my praise, her face now beaming with pride.

During the subsequent weeks, Alice continued to frequently visit the bar and began socializing with more deaf friends. However, she didn't pursue work. I asked her why. "I don't know," she would typically reply. "I don't like to work with hearing people. They ignore me or make fun of me. They treat me unfairly and discriminate against me. They look down on me because I'm hard-of-hearing. When I worked at the pizza restaurant, people didn't even talk to me! They talked about me behind my back! They acted as if I wasn't even there!"

It would have been easy to view Alice as somewhat paranoid, perhaps as projecting her own sense of inferiority on to others. Indeed that interpretation appeared to have some merit, as she was in line for a pay raise and advancement—hardly an obvious indication of discrimination. The mockery and belittling that she attributed to her coworkers also seemed to echo her own sense of inadequacy that she had alluded to earlier.

Moreover, it is a common experience for persons who have a significant hearing loss to feel anxious, intimidated and belittled as a result of being unable to adequately understand conversations in their social environment. Environmentally induced paranoia is, in large part, a natural consequence of being able to understand only a limited number of verbal and nonverbal social cues.[a] We fill in the blanks of what we don't understand, often in accordance with our subterranean fears that "people are talking about me." In this manner, conversational isolation provides fertile soil for us to project those disowned, negative, "shadow" parts of our self-esteem onto others.

Regardless of whether or not Alice imagined previous instances of ridicule and exclusion at the pizza parlor, it would be important to validate that they are at least frequently present in our prejudiced world. Members of any oppressed minority know too well the disquieting feeling that one is a "problem" in the eyes of the majority. As W. E. B. Du Bois wrote in 1903,

> Between me and the other world, there is ever an unasked question: unasked by some through feelings of delicacy; by others through the difficulty of rightly framing it... instead of saying directly, How does it feel to be a problem? they say, I know an excellent colored man in my town... Do not these Southern outrages make your blood boil? At these times I smile,

---

a. As is described in detail in Chapter 8, Overcoming Isolation and Despair, one's cognitive assumptions, attributions, and self-statements also play a large part in causing anxiety and paranoid sentiments.

or am interested, or reduce the boiling to a simmer, as the occasion may require. To the real question, How does it feel to be a problem? I answer seldom a word.[2]

I imagined that Alice had not only sensed this "unasked question" from the "other world" of her old job, she also sensed its answer. Neither were framed with delicacy, but were tinged with dehumanizing wrath. "How do you feel to be a problem to us? We don't care because you're subhuman, inferior, scum. We will therefore ignore you, not even talk to you."

In my view, Alice had been presented with another important life lesson, one beyond "don't park your car in tow zones": that even with sensitivity campaigns, the Americans with Disabilities Act, and other laws protecting the rights of disabled people, at least subtle discrimination and rejection will continue to occur. Many hearing people, in fact, *do* talk behind the backs of deaf/hard-of-hearing people; many ignore and avoid them; and many openly and maliciously denigrate them. The impact on one's assertiveness and self-esteem is potentially devastating. As Professor Tom Humphries, himself Deaf, noted, "Surrounded by powerful ideas of others that they were less than human, how could deaf–mutes conceive of themselves as anything more?"[3]

My task with Alice was to help her separate her own fears, fragile self-esteem and projections from the external reality that she may be someone's "problem." I asked her to tell me more about being made fun of and ignored at her old job.

"Everybody would talk and laugh with each other and make fun of me."

"How did you know they were making fun of you?"

"I just knew. I could tell."

"What would people do that you took to mean that they were making fun of you?"

"They were, that's all! They were talking and laughing at me. They looked toward me. I saw them!"

Versions of this exchange occupied most of the session. Finally, I asked Alice to rate her confidence about her interpretations. "Could they have looked at you for any other reason? Could they have laughed for any other reason? How do you know what they, in fact, were saying if you couldn't understand them?" But despite my trying to introduce reasonable doubt into Alice's attributions of blame, she remained steadfast in her belief that she was the object of their ridicule. It soon became clear that it was Alice's terror of being "a problem for the majority" without the security of her mother's comfort that kept her glued to her father's couch and out of the job market.

However, the environment at her father's house was anything but comfortable. A vicious cycle: her dad converses with someone; Alice interprets a verbal or nonverbal cue as derisive to her; she screams at her dad and goes to her room; her dad tries to console her, but with complicated words that she can neither lipread nor comprehend; Alice defends her position; Tom defends his position; her frustration escalates; his frustration escalates; and they go back to their respective corners, only to replay the same scene sooner or later. In this family context, she re-experienced the terror that had previously been limited to work and school.

One day Tom called me frantically to say that the cycle at home had changed for the worse. During one of their mutual escalations, Alice did not retreat in terror, but instead, smashed her bedroom window and threatened to throw the broken glass in his face. Within hours and with prodding from Tom's partner, he kicked Alice out of the house. Less than an hour after that, he changed the locks.

Several days later, Alice showed up for our scheduled appointment looking unkempt and bereft. "Your dad called me," I acknowledged to her. "What happened?"

"He got me mad. He wouldn't listen to me! He wouldn't get out of my room!"

"And what did you do?"

"I got so mad that I threw my chair at the window.... And he still wouldn't leave! And now he won't let me back home!" She paused and pounded her fist on her knee. "He kicked me out!" she screamed in pained outrage. "He should give me more time! I'm not ready to live on my own!"

Since Tom told her to leave, Alice was staying with a friend with whom, just one month ago, she had reestablished contact at the weekly bar gatherings. But she desperately wanted to go back home and felt infuriated and rejected by her dad, probably thinking that he favored his woman partner over her. Straight out of the W. E. B. Du Bois quotation, she undoubtedly felt like she was a problem to her father, much like she had felt like a problem to the hearing majority at work. Although she acknowledged that "I shouldn't have broken the window and threatened to throw the broken glass at my dad," in the same breath she gave greater emphasis to "he shouldn't have made me so mad!" Ultimately, she deemed the culpability as his, not hers.

I suggested that we invite her dad to join our next meeting so we could process what had happened. As she wasn't ready to live independently, I hoped that Tom would provide her with some support. Alice readily agreed to the joint meeting, probably viewing it as an opportunity to talk her dad into allowing her back home. At both of their requests, we scheduled a sign language interpreter.

There are moments when I feel old. One of those moments occurred two weeks later when I greeted Tom and Alice in my waiting room. I warmly shook Tom's hand and said I was sorry that our reunion was not on a happier occasion. He had obviously aged, now showing streaks of gray hair and wrinkles under his eyes. He looked somber. There was also a stiffness about his posture that I hadn't remembered noticing before. I imagined that he, too, felt old.

For the first time, I saw Alice's resemblance to her mother; both had striking deep facial features that seemed to mark their sensitivity to the world. Sadly, I once again found myself wishing that Nancy was alive and that she and her family were living happily ever after as planned. I shuddered to think what Nancy would have said if she were somehow watching the present family drama.

More flashbacks. There was a déjà vu quality to Alice smashing her window as I remembered Tom's initial outburst in my office, which I still codify as "the coffee incident." Enough reminiscing, we had work to do. Tom and Alice hadn't seen each other since the decisive incident, which occurred slightly over two weeks ago. Having had a brief premeeting session with the interpreter, I was ready to begin.[b] I beckoned them into my office.

Alice sat in her usual position on my couch, a ritual that I had long since imagined was a metaphor for the reason Tom had originally wanted me to see her. Oddly enough, Tom took the same seat that he had occupied during his visits with Nancy. Like father, like daughter. In sim-comm, Alice asked the interpreter to sit near her father. I took the remaining seat. The communication logistics, per Alice's request, were that she would sim-comm; I would sim-comm with her and use speech with Tom; and the interpreter would sign Tom's vocalizations.

However, I immediately found myself deliberately violating the agreement that I had made just seconds ago by using ASL, naturally without voice, to say "I would like to hear what goals both of you have for this meeting, what you want to accomplish. Who wants to start?" I wanted to "send" a special invitation for Alice to actively participate, as I predicted she would be the most reticent. The interpreter voiced my introduction so Tom would understand.

Tom, however, took the lead. "I'd just like to say very clearly to Alice that I'm willing and very much want to help her get on her feet. I don't want to take over her life so I need to hear from her exactly what kind of help, if any, she wants from me. I'm her dad and I love her." He then looked directly at Alice. "But I need to say—and I need to make this perfectly clear—that you coming back is definitely not, I repeat, *not,* an option."

---

b. Chapter 7, Beyond the Tug-of-War, describes the logistics of including interpreters in family therapy, including pre- and postmeetings.

"How about you, Alice? What do you want to have happen during this meeting with your dad?"[c]

"I'm sorry for breaking my bedroom window," she signed while the interpreter voiced. She looked down toward the floor and became silent.

"Thank you, Alice. I know you're sorry." Although Tom's appreciation seemed bonafide, his countenance reflected a discordant tenseness, perhaps because he knew what was coming next.

"But," Alice immediately added, "I want to come home. I'm not ready to go out on my own. You promised that I can stay with you for another year until I'm 25."

"That's not possible, Alice. I'm sorry."

"You promised." Her voice became a bit more desperate.

"I said it's impossible." His voice became a bit more firm.

"But—"

"No buts." Tom gave me a pleading look.

"Alice," I interjected, now taking my cue from Tom, "given that your dad's not going to let you come back home, maybe you could negotiate with him about what help he would be willing to give you."

"It's not fair, it's not fair!" she proclaimed, only to shrug her shoulders and again slump in the couch, seemingly engulfed by the weight of the world. Then she got a second wind. Not yet ready to give up bargaining for a postponement of the inevitable, she renewed her protests about the unfairness of her father's premature action, admonishing him for going back on his promise that she could live with him "until I turn 25." But in reaction to her dad's persistent refusals, her protests weakened and dissolved into sullenness.

"Alice, would you like to hear from your dad what kind of help he will give you?" I again asked.

She nodded her head unconvincingly.

---

c. Here, I used sim-comm, following Alice's lead. For more conceptually difficult dialogue with Alice, I switch to ASL, with the interpreter voicing for Tom.

Tom nevertheless began his part of the negotiations. He offered to help her move into an apartment; he would pay the first few months rent until she could find a job; he would cosign the lease. He would fund our individual therapy. He offered to meet with the vocational rehabilitation counselor with her. He offered to help pay for computer classes or any other kind of training that Alice and her vocational rehabilitation counselor felt would result in a job. He recited other possibilities. "Maybe you should go back to school, go to a community college, go to Gallaudet? You have a lot of choices, Alice. The world is yours."

Alice said nothing. She was immobilized by the complexities of her sudden emancipation.

"What are you going to do?" Tom asked again and again.

Alice shrugged her shoulders.

"You need to do something. You can't just do nothing. You need to call... You need to send out resumes. You need to..." Tom's face was getting redder and his voice was becoming louder.

"You said I could live with you longer. It's too soon to—"

"Alice, we had this talk! Now what are you going to do about..." After a few minutes, now Tom sank back and shrugged his shoulders, seemingly engulfed by the weight of Alice's passive refusal to participate in constructing her life. An endless, mutually frustrating cycle.

"Tom," I interrupted, "you must have had some experiences in your earlier life feeling scared, not knowing what to do, feeling overwhelmed with the world?" Images of Tom's previous workaholism and hiding came to mind.

Obviously feeling comfortable with my having given him an opening, he replied, "Of course, I have. Many times." He accentuated his message by several emphatic head nods. Now Alice perked up and she made eye contact with him.

"Would you tell your daughter some stories of when you felt like how she's probably feeling now? When in your life did you feel the most overwhelmed, scared, desperate?" I didn't realize what his answer would be, but in retrospect, it should have been obvious to me. As if Tom knew what I was driving at, he made anxious eye contact with me. I then realized his imminent answer.

"Go ahead," came my gut-level response. "Your daughter needs to know." An important, healing truth-telling process was happening. The story had to be told.

Now Tom looked at Alice lovingly with a vulnerability that I and perhaps Alice had never seen before. After a pause, he began, "It was when you had meningitis and were in the hospital. It was late at night. I still remember my utter terror and sadness when I found out. I was so scared and confused. I didn't know what to do, so I left and took a long walk. It was a nightmare, a horrible nightmare!" Tears came to all of our eyes.

"And your entire world caved in?" I volunteered, remembering the story that he had told me sitting in the same seat several years ago.

"Yes, absolutely. My whole entire world caved in, it sure did. I remember every detail as if it was yesterday." Before us, he once again relived that awful night.

To me the connection was obvious, but still had to be made explicit. "So maybe you know some of what Alice feels now? She finds herself in a world that is terribly frightening to her, one that she doesn't understand, one that represents *her* worst nightmare."

Tom nodded his head and looked at his scared daughter. "Alice," Tom said now in a more comforting voice, "I can understand how you feel. I remember other times in my life when..." He recounted several such instances, taking great pains to construct analogies that would do justice to every nuance of his experiences that he so desperately wished to share with her. He ended with "You must feel scared, intimidated, like the whole world's consuming you, eating you up..."

Out of the corner of my eye, I noticed the interpreter conveying the meaning of Tom's confusing English idiom of "eating you up." Like other skillfully executed art forms, I marveled how quickly and seemingly effortlessly she transformed the vocabulary, syntax, and idioms of his spoken English to a more conceptually based signing structure. Indeed, Tom naturally took the interpreter's presence for granted, almost forgetting that she was in the room. Although some say this is what is supposed to happen—that the interpreter should be invisible—here, I wanted the opposite: the interpreter should become *more* visible than ever. I wished to make accessible to Tom the several complex decisions that the interpreter was making. Then I could begin teaching him some principles of how to communicate more clearly with Alice.

"Tom, it's important that you know what the interpreter did to clarify your statement to Alice that 'I know how you feel. You must feel scared, intimidated, like the whole world's consuming you, eating you up.' She did something like "YOU FEEL WHAT? I KNOW. WORLD BIG, YOU SMALL. IDIOM: WORLD EAT YOU UP. MEAN WORLD SQUASH YOU. YOU SCARED. FEEL SMALL." This is an intervention that I sometimes use in family therapy in order to make linguistic issues more open to examination.[4] Naturally, the interpreter interpreted for Alice my impromptu attempt to gloss her ASL. As she and I had worked together many times before, she was not thrown off guard.

Now Tom looked both surprised and intrigued. I asked Alice "Would you tell your dad how often—at least what you're aware of—that you don't understand him?"

She needed no further prompting. Alice listed numerous instances of when "he kept talking and talking" and how "I would have no idea what you're talking about." Her recollections were not limited to face-to-face interactions; they also included their conversations on the TTY where "you go on and on." In this manner, environmentally induced paranoia, described earlier in the context of social groups, had been operative within her family. Her mild attentional disorder and dyslexia were further impediments.

"What are you more comfortable with: ASL or English?" I asked, remembering when Alice switched from sim-comm to ASL with me many sessions ago.

"I sort of go back and forth," she responded. "Sometimes for difficult stuff, ASL is easier. Like, I have no idea what 'eating you up' meant until she (the interpreter) interpreted it the right way. But most of the time, I like English."

We both thanked Alice for her disclosure. Tom added, now with a change of composure, that, "It was brave of you to tell me that. It took a lot of courage. I need to make sure you understand me."

"One way, it seems, that you can help your daughter is to make what you say accessible to her." He nodded his head. Although her stated preference was English, I reminded him that she benefited from ASL for "difficult stuff." I then spent some time explaining to Tom some very basic concepts of American Sign Language, such as time and place localization. I recommended that he take ASL classes. Although he responded affirmatively, his true intent remained unclear. Nonetheless, I was hopeful that the intervention of making the process of interpretation accessible to Tom would at least improve the quality of their communication.

It was time to add more stories to their dialogue that would provide Alice with a map from which to navigate in the world. Indeed, it is from our stories that we learn about life's lessons. The more varied our stories, the better. I didn't want the meningitis/Tom wandering through Boston story to be the primary illustration of Tom dealing with overwhelming anxiety, lest Alice feel somehow responsible and guilty for having been the cause of it. She would, of course, have no logical reason for feeling this way—she did not cause her own meningitis or her father's reaction to it—but human guilt and other emotions are often not based on logic.

"Tom, would you share with your daughter some other important lessons of life that you've learned so far, ones that you think would be particularly important for her to learn?"

He gave my request just a few seconds of thought, then blurted out his response as though he had been waiting for an appropriate opening. "Alice, probably one of the most important lessons I've learned is that life isn't always fair. I remember when I was once in line for a job promotion. I deserved it, I was promised it, and I counted on it. But then at the last minute, my boss gave the job to one of his family relatives. He got it instead of me."

"That's not fair!" exclaimed an incredulous Alice.

"Again, life isn't always fair," her dad replied.

I found myself recalling a sad moment when my then six-year-old daughter asked me what rape meant. My response was something like "it's when someone hurts someone else." She, too, responded with "But, Daddy, that's not fair!" I, too, responded with, "I know honey, but the world isn't always fair." With marked ambivalence, I would often take on the role of carefully bursting her bubble. There are many good things in this world, but one must be cautious of evil as well.

Tom was in a similar role with his daughter. In order to help her leave home and function more independently as a young adult, his parental task was to help break Alice's bubble of naive idealism about the inevitable goodness of humanity. He would become a catalyst for her to begin an important grieving process whereby she first acknowledges and eventually accepts that a segment of the world is unfair, racist, and oppressive. In my opinion, coming to terms with the delicate balance—the dialectic—of both accepting and confronting unfairness is an essential developmental milestone for any disabled person or member of an oppressed minority.

"What did you do when your boss didn't give you a raise?" a now more engaged Alice asked her dad.

"I was real, real angry about it for a long time. I remember running laps around the school track almost every night, just to work my anger off. And I had to spend a long time trying to figure out if there was something I did that caused me not to get promoted— whether or not it was my fault—or whether my boss was being unfair to me."

Alice nodded her head but it looked like something else was on her mind. I asked her what she was thinking.

Now looking directly at her dad, she asked, "Were you angry

when Mom died?"

Tom was taken aback by her apparently abrupt change of subject. But this time, Alice supplied the context. "Mom dying wasn't fair either, was it?"

Tom immediately shook his head and softened. "No sweetheart, Mom dying wasn't fair at all."

"Why did she have to die? There has to be a reason! There must be a reason!" Alice cried out and then she looked away. For an instant, I flashed back to what the Dalai Lama said about our obsession with finding clear reasons for everything. But now was not the time for pedagogy.

"Please go ahead," I said to her. I felt there was more to come.

"But you didn't seem to care," Alice tentatively remarked.

"What do you mean I didn't care?"

"I mean you don't care about what Mom said to do!"

"What do you mean?" Tom persisted.

"I mean that she told you to take care of me. And—"

"Alice, we've been through this. I'm trying to help you grow up! That's one important way I'm taking care of you! Besides, you're the one who threatened ME with the glass!" His voice now again became angry.

"Alice, you were going to say something?" I interjected, wishing to hear the end of her statement before Tom had interrupted her. I hadn't missed her change from the past tense to the present tense of "you don't care."

"You don't take care of her rose garden," she yelled.

A confused pause, dissipated by exasperation. "Her rose garden! What the hell does her rose garden have to do with anything!" Tom shouted.

"Let's find out," I said softly, also motioning with my hands for him to calm down and listen to Alice's answer. His question was reasonable although not inviting of an answer.

"You let her rose garden die. All her roses are dead. You let them die!" Alice, too, began to yell.

"But I moved! Her rose garden's at the old house. I don't own it anymore!"

"Hold on a minute, Tom. This is very important. I wonder if Alice views herself as another rose?" I then looked at Alice and signed in ASL an explanation of my tentative interpretation: namely that perhaps Tom letting the roses die out of neglect felt to her like he was letting her die out of neglect as well. Alice slowly nodded her head.

Tom also nodded his head, understanding the now obvious symbolism of roses. In a compassionate voice, he again explained to Alice that his goal was to help her grow up and become more independent, not to let her die "like a flower." She finally appeared to understand the distinction, but something was still left unsaid. Maybe it had to do with her mother.

"Alice, do you have any questions that you've been wanting to ask your dad about your mom?" I asked.

"Yeah. Did you love her?" came her hesitant inquiry.

"Yes, I did," Tom responded.

"Then why did you fight all the time?"

"It's a good but complicated question, sweetheart. I wasn't as mature then as I should have been. I had a temper. I remember the first time your mom and I were in Mike's office. Do you see that stain? (points to a part of my rug that has remnants of the "coffee incident") I actually flung coffee over the rug because I got so angry. I wasn't thinking."

Alice now looked compassionately both at her dad and the rug stain. She knew what it was like to lose her temper, to wrestle with the easily said but difficult challenge of coping with perceived unfairness, whether it occurs on the job, with one's spouse, or with one's parent. Then Alice made a final declaration of perhaps the ultimate act of unfairness that had been inflicted on her. "I'm sorry Mom's not here."

"I am, too," Tom said.

***

On a beautiful summer day, Tom picked up Alice for a Sunday drive. He drove several hours out of town through farm lands and countryside. Finally, he parked at a small shack amidst many orchids. It had been Nancy's favorite nursery.

Alice told me later that she didn't know why they were there. But Tom did. He bought a healthy looking rose bush, along with fertilizer and some new gardening tools. By mid-afternoon, they arrived at her dad's house and went to the backyard. It took them several hours to plant the bush. Little was said between them, not because of inadequate communication accessibility, but because there was simply no need for words.

A rose is a living object of sublime beauty. With proper soil, watering, nutrients, and care, the bush was sure to flourish. It would welcome the sun's rays and other acts of kindness; and it would tolerate storms, drought, and other acts of unkindness.

Tom never did take ASL classes. To this day, he often gets angry at Alice; and Alice often gets angry at him. But after these and other storms comes the sunshine. She is living with a roommate in an apartment for which Tom cosigned the lease. She got a job at a department store. More storms follow: A month ago, her car got towed again for the same reason as before. "I forgot," Alice lamented in my office. She was fired from her job because of consistent oversleeping. More sunshine: She is now taking computer classes at a nearby community college.

Some of life's lessons have to be presented to us several times before they are finally understood.

Alice and I continued to work together for approximately one year, with intermittent meetings with her father. We often focused on the critical task that Tom had brought up: to determine when one is victimized from when one abdicates one's own responsibility. Oversleeping was Alice's fault. The store insisting that she take customer orders on the telephone was their fault.

Amidst the sunlight and storms of Alice's and Tom's lives, they are sure to see each other regularly. Tom often takes her out to dinner and recently bought her some new clothes "for job interviews." But perhaps their most important ritual occurs without fail on Alice's birthday. On that special day, Alice and Tom visit the rose bush in his backyard. Sometimes for a few seconds, other times for several minutes, they stand in silence in front of it; then they exchange some banter about how well it's doing. Next, Tom gets out his gardening equipment that he shares with Alice. Finally, they complete their annual ritual of carefully watering, pruning and fertilizing the sacred bush. It is sure to produce beautiful roses.

Notes

1. His Holiness the Dalai Lama & Cutler, H.C. (1998). *The art of happiness.* New York, NY: Riverhead Books.
2. Dubois, W.E.B. (1903, reprinted in 1969). *The souls of black folk. Markham, Ontario: Penguin Books.*
3. Glickman, N. S., & Harvey, M.A. (1996). *Culturally affirmative psychotherapy with Deaf persons.* Mahweh, NJ: Lawrence Erlbaum.
4. Harvey, M.A. (1988). *Psychotherapy with deaf and hard-of-hearing persons: A systemic model.* Mahweh, NJ: Lawrence Erlbaum.

CHAPTER 10

Sharing the Wisdom of Old Age

Joan always followed her doctor's orders. Unlike my generation that prides itself for questioning authority, Joan didn't question Dr. Smith's request that she make an appointment with me. She arrived in my waiting room 10 minutes early.

We exchanged initial pleasantries. She confirmed that my directions to the office were clear and we agreed that the weather was a bit too humid. Joan looked her age of 71 years, with neatly combed white hair, thick-lensed glasses, and wearing a checkered, loose-fitting, slightly wrinkled dress. With some effort, she sat down on the straight-backed, least comfortable seat in my office, reporting that "my chiropractor said that's what I have to do." She then offered only a blank stare and waited for me to begin.

"How can I help?" came my usual opening question.

"Help with what?" came her response.

"With why you came."

"My doctor said I should make an appointment with you," Joan volleyed back.

"Do you know why?"

"No, I really don't. Dr. Smith gave me your phone number and told me to call you."

We were off to a slow start. Wishing to speed things up a bit, I said to her, "Dr. Smith feels that you may be depressed or that something else might be bothering you."

"Dr. Smith is a wonderful man," Joan responded, now with a bit more enthusiasm. "He's a very good doctor and always has time for me."

"That's nice," came my response. So far we had used up 5 minutes; 45 minutes to go.

"Do you agree with him?" I finally asked.

"About what?"

"About feeling depressed!" Forty-four minutes to go.

"It's sweet of him to be concerned about me. But no, I don't feel depressed."

"I see."

"You see what?" she asked quite seriously.

"I see that you don't feel depressed. But—if it's okay with you— let me read Dr. Smith's referral note about you. Okay?"

"Of course."

"It says 'This 71-year-old woman has been widowed for six years; is losing both her hearing and vision; and, within the past few years, has had two hip replacements and has undergone open heart surgery.'" I then told her that her doctor requested that I help her "better deal with these losses as she is markedly withdrawn and is exhibiting other depressive symptoms."

"It's nice of him to be so concerned. He's a very good doctor, a nice man," she again stated.

"I know; and he takes a lot of time with you," I purposely smiled. My conscious intent was to introduce some levity into our prolonged introduction; but admittedly, my response was more sarcastic than intended. It undoubtedly reflected my growing impatience on the heels of what had been a long day. The referring physician's assessment seemed obvious to me but not to Joan.

She smiled and retorted with "That's right, he takes a lot of time, just as I had told you before." Maybe she was also getting impatient with me?

When in doubt reach for the chart. I had a standard diatribe of history—taking questions—a necessary but perhaps premature ritual. Necessary because it would guide treatment; premature because it was done in the service of imposing my own structure, perhaps too early in our relationship. Before I could complete even the first question—"What is your birthday?"—Joan interrupted with "Is that a picture of your daughter over there on your wall?"

"Uh yes," I replied now putting down my pad and pen. "But she's only three in that picture; now she's nine years old." I found myself feeling a bit negligent.

Sure enough, she immediately asked "Why haven't you put up a new picture of her?"

I laughed defensively. After a few "umms," I said that it's on my "to do list."

"I update my pictures every year," Joan proclaimed with obvious pride.

"I should do the same," I again admitted.

"Here, I'll show you some of mine!" Joan took out her wallet-sized photograph binder. "This is my grandson. He..."

I had unwelcome flashes of my grandmother showing me her endless array of photos, complete with an eternity of excruciatingly boring details. However, with Joan, maybe this ordeal would be a conversational opener.

"...Tommy, he's eight years old and was just in a school play," Joan continued. "Here's his sister, Diane. You can see her braces, see? She just got them and for the first night, they hurt her but it got better. She loved taffy so much but now..." Joan's face beamed, just like my grandmother's.

After 20 or so pictures and 40 minutes of stories, I managed to get the date of her birthday. (Good material for her chart). She also agreed to schedule another appointment. In preparation, I found a more recent photograph of my daughter to hang on my wall. I also hung a photo of my other daughter. Luckily, Joan hadn't asked me whether I have other children and, if so, why their pictures had never even made it to my office.

Sure enough, a week later, upon inspecting both photographs, Joan's first comment was "So you have two daughters?"

"I do," I muttered.

"They're beautiful," she remarked.

"Well, thank you!" I sighed, relieved that Joan had let me off the hook. However, I then noticed that she had placed five foot-high stacks of albums on the floor in front of her. "Are those more albums of your children?" I asked with an attempt to hide my trepidation.

Her instantaneous and enthusiastic nod came as no surprise. Thank God she only has five children, I thought. A quick calculation: Five times roughly 50 pictures per child equals 250 pictures, each with a minute or so of narrative equals 250 minutes, or 4 hours and 10 minutes.

Per my prediction, Joan spent the next several sessions showing me various photographs of her five children, taken at different camera angles, at assorted locations, with and without dog or cat, in front of a bush, beside a bush, in back of a bush, etc. I nodded politely after each photograph, so much so that I imagined my head becoming loose on my neck.

Now for the good news: this ritual did indeed provide the context for her to share with me parts of her life story that she could never have shared via traditional history-taking. Joan told me about the frequent get-togethers the whole family would have with all five adult children, their spouses and the assembly of grandchildren. Typically, even some neighborhood kids would join in the fun festivities: hot dogs on the grill, "tons of sugar," volleyball, swimming in a huge pool, horseshoes. With a tone of dignified pride, Joan told me that "when I'm not taking pictures, I always sit in a seat reserved for me by the shallow end of the pool."

"Here's a picture of my daughter, Barbara," Joan continued. "She..." Barbara was a frequent feature of the family photographs marathon with significantly more photos and associated narrative than the rest of her children. I asked about their relationship.

"Out of the bunch, she worries about me the most," Joan reported. "She almost always comes to my doctors' appointments with me; and, in the old days, she used to call them no less than once a week to keep them up to date about my condition. Now she faxes them letters instead."

"I feel left out," I smirked. "No messages, no faxes, nothing!"

"She doesn't know about you," Joan quickly responded in a comforting voice.

"Why not? She knows about all the others," I smiled.

Joan smiled back. Then she got serious and said meekly, "I've never been to a shrink before."

"And?" I beckoned.

"And I don't know what she'd say."

"What do you think she might say?"

"That I'm off my rocker and on my way to a loony bin," Joan laughed, but this time unconvincingly. Going to a "shrink" was clearly not acceptable within her social network.

"You're very much *on* your rocker," I responded. "But people are worried about you being depressed; Barbara, your doctor and probably many others." For the remainder of our session, we discussed how Barbara "always" worries and how she sacrifices too much of her family life in order to case manage Joan's medical care. As Joan was about to leave, she blurted out somewhat provocatively that "Barbara's been dying to know where I've been for the past few Wednesdays at noon."

"Why don't you invite her to our meeting? We could show her that you're not loony tunes and help her stop worrying so much."

Joan let out a chuckle, saying "Oh, I don't know about that" and bid me good bye.

A surprise: The following Wednesday at noon brought Joan and Barbara to my waiting room. She looked like her many pictures—a miniature version of her mother, bright and alert but with furrows under her eyes. She carried a loose-leaf note book with an attached pen, apparently for any note-taking opportunities. Joan introduced me as "Dr. Harvey, my shrink."

"I've been called worse," I smiled, while shaking Barbara's hand and beckoning the two of them into my office.

Barbara had brought a portable FM system that Joan then hooked up to her hearing aid. We would pass the microphone to each other. I opted to begin with what had occupied center stage in Joan's photograph albums: the family gatherings. They obviously held great meaning for her; and, judging from what she had told me about Barbara's concern, I predicted they would provide a good conversation opener.

"Joan told me all about your wonderful family get-togethers."

"They're wonderful for all of us," Barbara quickly responded, "but not for my mother. I've been really concerned about her for a very long time and I'm glad she's finally seeing a therapist."

I ascertained that Joan understood what Barbara had said. "Why don't you think the get-togethers are wonderful for your mother?" I then asked Barbara.

"No matter what's going on, she always has the same expression on her face. She's lost in a world all her own, like she's in a cocoon. I know she can't understand any of the conversations around her even with her hearing aids!"

"And what happens when you or other family members suspect that she can't participate in the conversation?"

"Every once in a while, someone goes up to her and summarizes what has been said in the previous hour or so. Other times, I feel so sorry for her that I summarize verbatim what everyone's saying around her. But in either case, all she does is nod her head and say something like 'that's nice' or 'I'm glad you're having a good time.'"

Barbara continued her perceptive account. "When we continue to explain more details of the conversation to Mom, or perhaps to tell her a story of our own, her eyes begin to glaze over. She has little or no idea of what's being said. Maybe to spare our feelings or to save face—I really don't know—she acts as if she understands. But it doesn't work. It frustrates everybody."

This is a commonly described scenario of families in which there is a hard-of-hearing or deaf member. As Barbara continued to tell her story of why her mother was the way she was, Joan's eyes did indeed glaze over and she became very quiet, only nodding her head at seemingly random intervals. I imagined hooking up the word-count tool from my word processing software to somehow count the number of words Barbara and Joan spoke. The count would undoubtedly be at least a 100:1 ratio in favor of Barbara. Somehow in the presence of her daughter—who was obviously loving and concerned—Joan surrendered her voice and/or Barbara unwittingly stole it. Love does funny things to people.

"So who in the family is able to engage her the most?" I finally asked.

In response to her shrugging her shoulders, I repeated the question. After some thought, Barbara replied, "Well, I guess she does better with the kids. I don't know exactly why but she comes out of her shell with her grandchildren." Barbara shook her head and smiled, perhaps reflecting both her own frustration and her awe at the children's ability to access their grandmother.

"They don't even have a college degree and they can easily do what all of you can't?" I teased.

"Looks that way, doesn't it?" Barbara smiled. She had not given this phenomenon much thought until now.

"I wonder what their secret is," I asked, trying not to be obviously provocative. When no immediate response was forthcoming, I turned to Joan and asked her what she talks about with her grandchildren. She smiled and said simply, "Oh, they like to hear stories."

It appeared that the grandchildren were the first to figure out how to get their grandmother out of her "self-imposed cocoon." Apparently, they would ask grandma to tell her life's story. "Tell me about what kind of dog you had as a kid"; "Tell me when you went to Italy"; "Tell me about mom when she..."; and so on. I imagined that these prompts were a sort of on–off switch for Joan. Once engaged with any version of "tell me about," she would share detailed, vivid, passionate stories, undoubtedly, I thought, often accompanied by photographs. Barbara also reported that her mom's countenance would change from a kind of catatonic, somnambulistic withdrawal to a vibrant, entertaining story-teller. I had already witnessed this transformation in my office.

I asked Barbara to use the "tell me about" technique with her mother right now, here in the office.

With her jaw clenched, she grunted impatiently to Joan, "Tell me about what you're thinking when you're just sitting there by the pool every time you come over the house! You can't be happy!"

"A good beginning, I suppose. But that sounds like an indictment, a question that your mother shouldn't answer without her attorney present. Ask the question from a position of child-like curiosity. Ask your mom to tell you a story."

"A story about what?" Barbara asked somewhat incredulously.

"A story that you'd like to hear, perhaps for the first time, or maybe one that you'd like to hear again. Your mom has told you stories, right?"

It was a bit of a struggle to help Barbara honor her mother as a storyteller. Perhaps that's why it had come so easily for the grandchildren; they didn't know so much or think that they should be helpful. Instead, they wished and expected only to hear stories from their entertaining, wise, old grandmother.

After a pause and some awkward shifting in her chair, Barbara's demeanor became softer. She looked at her mother hesitantly and said, "Tell me about Dad."

Six years ago, Joan's husband of over 45 years had dropped dead one afternoon while they were walking their dog. Although she had incurred many health-related losses, the most devastating loss by far was James. Their last walk together seemed like only yesterday. She could easily recall what they were wearing, their conversation, the weather and even that they were going to rent an old Alfred Hitchcock movie that evening.

Joan's eyes welled up, as did Barbara's and mine. A painful pause. This time it was Joan who broke the silence by saying, matter-of-factly, "You know, Barbie, I still talk to him every night at dinner." For several years, she had regularly cooked James's favorite chicken dish, talked to him in the evenings and bid him good night. A shield against loneliness. I thought of a scene in Alfred Hitchcock's *Rear Window* of the widow entertaining imaginary men in her apartment.

I felt pity for Joan and a deep terror of what may someday be in store for me—to entertain imaginary people in my home. A quotation by Cicero. "As I give thought to the matter, I find four causes for the apparent misery of old age; first, it withdraws us from active accomplishments; second, it renders the body less powerful; third, it deprives us of almost all forms of enjoyment; fourth, it stands not far from death."[1] No wonder Barbara hadn't wanted to hear her mother's stories. No wonder I had originally reached so quickly for her chart. No wonder I was relieved that our time was up.

I needed to read more uplifting descriptions of old age. They would be found in a book by psychoanalyst and octogenarian Erik Erikson entitled *Vital Involvement in Old Age*. Erikson's premise, "In old age a human being must not only confront nonbeing but also face the final maturation of what we may call an existential identity."[2] It sounded right, even erudite enough to use in an upcoming lecture on human development. But I had little idea of what it meant.

Both Joan and Barbara returned for a second visit, ostensibly for Barbara to keep informed about her mother's progress. This time I began the session by reading Erickson's quotation. Barbara and I volunteered some academic-sounding verbiage that Joan correctly labeled as "hogwash." Joan knew exactly what Erikson meant, although she had never read his writings. As a preliminary hint, she offered a recollection. "Five years ago—a year after Jim died—I got dentures; three years ago, I had two hip replacements; a year ago, I had open heart surgery and got a pacemaker; and, three months ago, I got fitted for two hearing aids. Pretty soon, I'll have 'Made in Japan' stamped on me!"

She laughed and so did I. But I didn't know what I was laughing about. Barbara looked confused as well. "What do you mean?" I had to ask.

"With all these artificial devices in me, how do you think I know it's still me?" Joan asked.

"How *do* you know that you're really you?" I asked back. An odd phrasing to be sure, but I couldn't find a better alternative.

"Sure, I have a pacemaker in me that was made by someone else but it's *my* pacemaker. Sure, I just got two hearing aids made by someone else, but they're *mine!* Same with my hips, same with my dentures. These things give me life; they're part of me!"

This time it was Barbara who asked the bottom-line question. "But Mom, how do figure out what's you and what's not you?" Barbara recoiled as if she had asked either an offensive or stupid question.

Her mom, however, gave an immediate reply. "Sweetheart, I know it's me because of my memories! I've had many adventures," Joan smiled. "I remember when..."

A long story ensued. Although she had left her photograph albums at home, she related a tapestry of images, of dialogues, all blended together to bring the rich odyssey of her life into the present, before our eyes. Joan wasn't simply recounting her experiences, she recreated them for us. Joan also seemed to be acknowledging to herself the insights and wisdom she had to offer us, even to the point of insisting that we listen. I felt privileged, extremely honored to be in the presence of this wise, old grandma. Barbara, too, seemed impressed. We sat there and smiled knowingly at each other.

Her confronting "nonbeing" and struggling to forge an existential identity all seemed so natural to her. It was as if she proclaimed, "I am what I experience; I'm *not* the summation of bodily organs." Again, she intuitively understood another insight by Erikson. "Wisdom is detached concern with life itself, in the face of death itself. It maintains and learns to convey the integrity of experience, in spite of decline of bodily and mental functions."[3]

I privately wondered, however, whether one comes to appreciate the integrity of experience, not in spite of, but *because of* the decline of bodily functions. The progressive insertions of artificial devices into Joan's body and her imminent nonbeing—her death—catalyzed her existential crisis. It seemed a cruel but universal truism that often we human beings can truly value and appreciate something only when it is about to be taken away.

Joan had not only taken her share of the conversation but, more importantly, had given Barbara and I a glimpse of her emerging wisdom, of her odyssey of growing old. Although Barbara had heard the story of her dad's death many times before, she had never before borne witness to how her mom had learned to *reconcile* that loss, as well as a host of others, through her rich "integrity of experience." This time I was sorry it was time to stop. I bid mother and daughter a warm good-bye.

It was Joan who began our next individual meeting. "Dr. Harvey, tell me how you feel when you wake up in the morning."

"Depends if it's a workday or weekend," I replied half-jokingly.

"How does it feel to wake up on a workday?" she persisted, not about to let me off the hook.

"Let's see, I look at the clock, get in the shower... and drive to work."

"That's what you *do!* I thought you psychologists talk a lot about feelings. I asked you how do you *feel?*"

"I don't know. Tired, I run through in my head what I have to do that day—"

"Never mind," she interrupted. "You're not answering my question. I'll tell you how *I* feel: grateful to see the next day, happy to be alive, enjoying the breeze from the window. The sky reaches out and touches me, and I touch back; I sense a beautiful, knowing presence, something larger than the sky, larger than the sun and breeze. I stop and behold it all; and I pray." She sat perfectly still, but her mind left my office. With a flushed face, she had the same distant look in her eyes that she had during our first meeting, but now I understood more its origins: in psychological terms, a dissociative state; in theological terms, a religious experience.

Joan was attempting to teach me about her spiritual love affair with the universe. I thought of psychologist Jon Kabat-Zinn's reflection, "Perhaps ultimately, spiritual simply means experiencing wholeness and interconnectedness directly, seeing that individuality and the totality are interwoven, that nothing is separate or extraneous. If you see in this way, then everything becomes spiritual in its deepest sense. Doing science is spiritual. So is washing the dishes."[4]

Her spiritual love affair had been her carefully guarded secret. Its clues were limited to blank stares, withdrawal and, in her internist's words, "other depressive symptoms." What were the effects of her keeping what might be called her "rendezvous with God" so private? My mind flashed to several spouses in treatment who were having extramarital affairs. Indeed *any* private rendezvous—although from a distance may seem romantic and exhilarating—often leaves one feeling lonely and depressed afterward. People need people. I now wondered why she kept her spiritual rendezvous so private.

"Why do you just sit there at family parties?" I asked her again.

"What else should I do? Everyone's talking about gibberish; most of its boring to me and it's all muffled and distorted anyway!" She sat back in resignation.

"But aren't you lonely? Isolated? You have so much to offer!"

Almost in a whisper, Joan responded, "No one cares." Her face dropped toward the floor.

"No one cares?"

"I'm just an old lady." The room suddenly felt still; the air, heavy.

"You *are* an old lady," I affirmed in a deliberately playful way. Her faced perked up and she returned a confused smile. "Joan, you're teaching me about that which has terrified me and frankly continues to do so. Old age, losing my health and my organs, losing my senses, my family, my friends. At least intellectually, I can sort-of begin to understand the spiritual wisdom that you've achieved and how you may feel different than many others around you. Yes, you're an old lady who has a lot of wisdom to offer us younger folk who talk 'hogwash.'"

"And what is that wisdom exactly, Dr. Harvey?" she asked sarcastically or inquisitively (I wasn't sure which).

"How you define the value of your existence. How you can reconcile the opposites of feeling more human even though your body's falling apart. How you're able to feel more alive than you've ever felt as you stare death smack in the face. I really don't know what I'm talking about, Joan, as I haven't been there yet. But you're there! And you have a lot to teach us!" By this time I was beginning to yell.

Joan sat motionless and was quiet for a moment with a contemplative look on her face. Then in a soft, slow, compassionate voice, she asked me, "Dr. Harvey, do you love your children?"

"More than I can tell you," I replied instantly.

"Then why, when I first met you, did you not have their pictures on your wall?"

Stunned by her simple but painful question, I sat motionless. This time it was me who looked downward. "I didn't make time to do it," was my feeble justification.

Joan gazed straight into my eyes and gave a sage response. "I make time for those important things. That's how I know I'm alive."

A long silence ensued, as her words echoed through my soul.

That night, my kids probably thought I had too hard a day or was losing my marbles. Instead of my ritual of policing the completion of their homework, I said that it wasn't important and that I would write a note to their teachers. At my beckoning, they dressed up in beautiful clothes—dresses that I had bought them several weeks before—and posed for over an hour while I took so many pictures as to rival Joan's photo collection. Someday my kids will be gone, off living their own lives with their spouses and kids. And someday I will die. Their homework could wait, for at least a day.

The next week, I showed all the photos to Joan—the different poses (serious, happy, pensive, etc.)—with various camera angles, backgrounds, and other photographic nuances that only a professional or proud parent would understand. She politely endured the exhibition, nodding frequently so much that I imagined her head becoming loose on her neck.

Afterward, I thanked her for teaching me a lesson that I regularly forget and relearn: to cherish what is really important and, in the popular vernacular, "not sweat the small stuff." I added that we adults are frequently more resistant to learning this lesson than are children. I also commented that there are "a lot of resistant students in our world." Joan thought for a moment and nodded her head.

It was time to end our session (my photos had taken up most of the hour). We stood up and Joan abruptly gave me a hug. It was then that I noticed her tears. As she left, she whispered, "Thank you. I know what I need to do."

At our next meeting, Joan brought in an article she had come across by Betty Friedan, the originator of the phrase "feminine mystique" to describe our cultural conspiracy against women.[5] Joan took almost the full hour to explain how Friedan, now almost 80 years old, believes that many people succumb to the "rocking chair model" of old age and that this "age mystique" is every bit as oppressive and blighting of human possibility as sexism.

As she finished her lecture and got up to leave, I asked her whether she just wanted to share with me her newly discovered passion or to avoid being captive to more pictures of my daughters. She smiled and said, "Both."

***

A couple of weeks later, I got a message from Barbara on my answering machine. It seemed that Joan continued to maintain exclusive rights on her chair at the shallow end of the pool during subsequent family gatherings. However, now she no longer resigned herself to sitting silently by herself. She not only insisted on telling more stories, but she had taken to admonishing the "endless, meaningless chatter"; that her kids talk only about clothes, dieting, investments, computer gadgets, or idle gossip; and that most importantly, "there are better ways to use one's precious time left on earth."

Barbara ended her message by saying that she was pleased. But I detected a touch of ambivalence.

Joan makes an appointment with me every six months or so, reportedly to find out how I'm doing. She regularly inspects, not my diplomas or licensure status, but whether the photographs of my children are up to date. I have come to envy Joan, certainly not because of her declining bodily functions that will imminently betray her, but because she is fundamentally more alive than me. I have a lot to learn from her in the short time that is left for us.

Notes

1. Bennett, C.E. (Ed.) (1990). *Cicero: On old age.* Wauconda, IL: Bolchazy-Carducci.

2. Erikson, E.H., Erikson, J.M., & Kivnick, H.Q. (1986). *Vital involvement in old age.* New York: Norton.

3. Erikson, E.H., Erikson, J.M., & Kivnick, H.Q. (1986). *Vital involvement in old age.* New York: Norton.

4. Kabat-Zinn, J. (1994). *Wherever you go there you are: Mindfulness meditation in everyday life.* New York: Hyperion.

5. Simon, R. (1998). Betty Friedan takes on the age mystique. *Family Therapy Networker, 22*(4), 40–47.

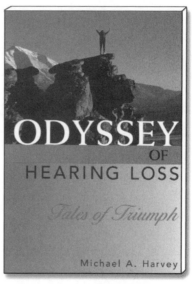
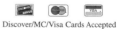
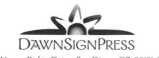